PRAISE FOR *DESCARTES' BABY*

"Paul Bloom has a gift for explaining the science of mental development, making it relevant to our everyday lives and to the latest scientific research. This book will excite a new generation of readers. In Bloom's hands, the sober science comes alive."
—Simon Baron-Cohen, Professor of Developmental Psychopathology
and author of *The Essential Difference*

"The twenty-first century was marked by the unveiling of the human genome. The twenty-second century will be marked by the discovery of how this chemical package creates human nature. If you are as impatient as I am for a glimpse of the ingredients that went into making us the knowing species, then treat yourself to Paul Bloom's wonderful book *Descartes' Baby*. It is a carefully argued, richly insightful, and deeply satisfying exploration of how and what we know about the physical, social and spiritual world."
—Marc Hauser, Ph.D., Co-Director,
Mind, Brain & Behavior Program, Harvard University

"[Bloom's] prose abounds with lively examples from conceptual art, contemporary fiction and his own child-rearing observations. The result is a delightful and humane study that makes rewarding reading for those interested in cognitive psychology's broader implications."
—*Publishers Weekly*

"Bloom's underlying philosophical aims are profound. He wishes to explain how notions such as morality, humour, art and identity are aspects of the human condition."
—London *Times*

"Paul Bloom's *Descartes' Baby: How the Science of Child Development Explains What Makes Us Human* manages to lift some weighty concepts with a lightness of touch. It's genuinely thoughtful and thought-provoking, rather than some wearingly trivial pop psychology book about how cute babies are."
—*Observer*

"[Bloom] succeeds in making the minds of children—who can seem exceedingly tedious to those not currently raising any—a fascinating place to spend a few hours."
—*Seed* Magazine

"In this thought-provoking book, Bloom posits that children are natural dualists, instinctively understanding the world as divided into two categories: physical objects and minds with intentions. . . . Readers new to the study of psychology, as well as students and scholars, will find much to spark further interest and research. Recommended for public and academic libraries."
Library Journal

D1246202

DESCARTES' BABY

How the Science of
Child Development Explains
What Makes Us Human

જ

PAUL BLOOM

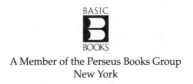

BASIC
BOOKS

A Member of the Perseus Books Group
New York

For Karen

Hardcover edition first published in 2004 by Basic Books,
A Member of the Perseus Books Group

Paperback edition first published in 2005 by Basic Books

The Library of Congress has catalogued the hardcover edition as follows:

Bloom, Paul, 1963-
    Descartes' baby : how the science of child development explains what
makes us human / Paul Bloom.
        p.   cm.
    Includes bibliographical references and index.
    ISBN 0-465-00783-X (hc)
    1. Cognition.   2. Child psychology.   I. Title.

BF311.B555 2004
153—dc22

2003022387

ISBN 0-465-00786-4 (pbk)

05 06 07 / 10 9 8 7 6 5 4 3 2 1

CONTENTS

Since the eighteenth century, there has been in circulation a curious story about Descartes. It is said that in later life he was always accompanied in his travels by a mechanical life-sized female doll, which, we are told by one source, he himself had constructed "to show that animals are only machines and have no souls." He had named the doll after his illegitimate daughter, Francine, and some versions of events have it that she was so lifelike that the two were indistinguishable. Descartes and the doll were evidently inseparable, and he is said to have slept with her encased in a trunk at his side. Once, during a crossing over the Holland Sea some time in the early 1640s, while Descartes was sleeping, the captain of the ship, suspicious about the contents of the trunk, stole into the cabin and opened it. To his horror, he discovered the mechanical monstrosity, dragged her from the trunk and across the decks, and finally managed to throw her into the water. We are not told whether she put up a struggle.

—Stephen Gaukroger,
Descartes: An Intellectual Biography

PREFACE

Sex with dead animals is disgusting. Someone slipping on a banana peel can be wildly funny. Killing babies is wrong. Splashes of paint on a canvas can be a work of art. Your body will change radically as you age, but you will remain the same person. And when you die, your soul may live on.

There are people who lack these basic notions, such as psychopaths who commit horrific acts without the slightest twinge of conscience, or severely autistic children, who have no understanding that other people have thoughts and emotions. But these unusual cases just prove the rule that notions such as morality, humor, art, and personal identity are aspects of the normal human condition.

How can we best explain this? Some scholars argue that these human characteristics are evolutionary adaptations that are hard-wired into babies' brains. Others see them as the product of culture, independent of biology and genetics, best explained in terms of historical and social processes. But I think a better explanation comes from the work of Charles Darwin. In *The Descent of Man* and *The Expression of the Emotions in Man and Animals,* Darwin proposed that many mental abilities emerged through natural selection—they arose through the reproductive advantages that they gave to our ancestors. But he was also clear that many uniquely human traits are not themselves adaptations. They are the by-products of adaptations—biological accidents.

I will explore Darwin's approach here. In particular, I will suggest that humans have evolved a certain way of thinking about people and objects. We see the world along the lines proposed by René Descartes, the father of modern philosophy.

Descartes was fascinated by the automata of his time, such as the hydraulically controlled robots at the French Royal Gardens that moved in realistic ways, acting as if angry or modest. He believed the bodies of humans and animals to be nothing more than particularly intricate machines. But for people—unlike for nonhumans, whom Descartes described as "beast-machines"—there is a crucial distinction between *res extensa,* our physiological machinery, and *res cogitans,* which is our selves, our minds. We use our bodies to experience and act on the world, but we ourselves are not physical things. We are immaterial souls.

We can explain much of what makes us human by recognizing that we are natural Cartesians—dualistic thinking comes naturally to us. We have two distinct ways of seeing the world: as containing bodies and as containing souls. These two modes of seeing the world interact in surprising ways in the course of the development of each child, and in the social context of a community of humans they give rise to certain uniquely human traits, such as morality and religion.

The effect that our dualism has on how we think and feel is illustrated by the epigraph that begins this book. There are different versions of this tale. Some have it that Descartes created the robot out of grief after what he described as the greatest sorrow of his life: the death of his daughter, Francine, at the age of five. Others claim that Descartes never had a human daughter, just this mechanical doll, born out of his fascination with automata. But the stories all end the same way, with the horror of the sea captain and the destruction of the machine.

There is something that many find disturbing, even revolting, about the notion of a soulless body, a purely physical creature that acts as though it were a person. This reaction is worrisome, given the scientific consensus that Descartes was mistaken. Modern science tells us that the conscious self arises from a purely physical brain. We do not have immaterial souls; we are material beings, no less than the "monstrosity" drowned by the captain. We are Descartes' babies.

I begin by laying out the foundations of infants' mental development, showing that before they can speak or walk or control their bowels, babies see the world as containing both physical things, which are governed by principles such as solidity and gravity, and immaterial minds, which are driven by emotions and goals. Babies are natural-born dualists.

Chapters 2 and 3 show how our duality of perception shapes how we make sense of the artificial and natural world. It helps explain why even children are prone to believe in a divine creator. And it explains some mysteries concerning our appreciation of art, such as why we take so seriously the difference between a forgery and the original and what distinguishes a work of art from everything else.

I then turn to how our intuitive dualism underlies our feelings toward other people. Chapter 4 concerns the emergence of moral sentiments in babies and children, and chapter 5 discusses the growth of the "moral circle," the universe of beings encompassed by our developed moral sense. I present a theory of the emergence of a uniquely human morality, and discuss how certain forces can enhance, nourish, and solidify our evolved moral sense, transforming it in profound ways.

Chapter 6 reviews the fascinating literature on disgust. While emotions such as empathy can expand the moral circle, feelings of disgust can diminish it, causing us to see people as creatures without moral worth. This chapter ends with a discussion of slapstick humor, which, surprisingly, also rests on an appreciation of the body/soul duality.

The final two chapters concern our spiritual beliefs. Chapter 7 explores how our intuitive dualism shapes how children and adults think about personal consciousness and life after death. And chapter 8 explores our belief in spiritual beings, such as trees that can remember conversations and the God of the Old Testament. I conclude with a discussion of how our commonsense dualism meshes with a scientific conception of reality.

I first became interested in these issues about eight years ago, after hearing Paul Rozin talk about his research on disgust. Although my primary interest at the time was the study of language development, the topic intrigued me. When I joined the Psychology Department at Yale University in 1999, I taught a graduate seminar called "Bodies and Souls," and it was there that the idea for this book began to emerge.

Yale University has provided a stimulating and supportive environment to pursue this work, and I owe a lot to my colleagues. I am especially grateful to my long-suffering graduate students, who have been supportive and helpful even as I repeatedly shifted the focus of our lab meetings away from their own substantive research in child development onto topics such as modern art and necrophilia.

Steven Pinker gave me some excellent advice when I was mulling over whether to begin this project. I also benefited greatly from the encouragement and support of my agent, Katinka Matson.

I am grateful as well to those who shared their expertise with me on a variety of topics: Woo-Kyoung Ahn, Renée Baillargeon, Jesse Bering, Amy Campbell, Susan Carey, Elizabeth Cashdan, Geoffrey Cohen, Deborah Fried, Sharmin Ghaznavi, James Grossman, Paul Harris, Carl Johnson, Serene Jones, Donna Lutz, Joseph Mahoney, Melissa Allen Preissler, Peter Salovey, Brian Scholl, Michelle Sternthal, and Rob Wilson.

Several friends, former students, and colleagues—and in a few cases, people I have never met—took the time to provide detailed comments on drafts of different chapters. I thank Pascal Boyer, Cheryl Browne, Gil Diesendruck, Jonathan Haidt, Deborah Kelemen, Jerrold Levinson, Barbara Malt, Lori Markson, Gregory Murphy, David Pizarro, Paul Rozin, Laurie Santos, Peter Singer, Karen Wynn, and Ed Zigler. I am particularly grateful to Frank Keil and

Susan Gelman, who both provided extensive feedback on several chapters. My greatest debt here is to my editor at Basic Books, Jo Ann Miller, who gave me advice at every stage of this project and who greatly improved the final manuscript with her detailed and penetrating comments.

The support of my family—in Connecticut, Quebec, Massachusetts, Ottawa, Texas, and Saskatchewan—mattered more to me than they will ever know. My sons, Max and Zachary, kept me aware that abstract theories have to apply to real children—and ensured that the years that I wrote this book were among the happiest of my life. Most of all, I thank my wife, Karen Wynn. Karen has been incredibly supportive, and every idea in this book has been shaped by my discussions with her. I would not have completed *Descartes' Baby* without Karen's kindness, her brilliance, and her love. I dedicate it to her.

PART I

FOUNDATIONS

1

MINDREADERS

The child is father to the man.
—Wordsworth

WHAT DOES IT take to win the World Series of Poker? It is not just luck. Hundreds of players enter the competition, each one with a ten-thousand-dollar stake, and year after year, pretty much the same characters end up at the final table. It is not that they have any special knowledge. The rules of the game, no-limit Texas hold 'em, can be explained to a novice in less than an hour, and anyone with patience and a good head for numbers can learn the percentages. Certainly some elusive quality of character comes into play: you need to know when to hold them and know when to fold them, know when to walk away and know when to run. But this is not what makes the winners special.

Al Alvarez, a poet and poker player, answers the question nicely when he says of a master gambler that he doesn't play the cards—he plays the other players. Those who win the World Series are superb *mindreaders*. As Alvarez says, "One of the many gifts that separates the professionals from the amateurs is the ability to read their opponents' hands with uncanny accuracy from the tiniest clues: timing, position, the way their fingers move their chips or their eyes flicker, even the pulse beat in their neck."

Poker professionals must be not only adept at reading the minds of others but also capable of obscuring their own thoughts. They must act so that their opponents are either at a total loss when it comes to figuring out their mental states or—even better—mislead their opponents into making false inferences about their mental state, as when they successfully bluff, or convince someone that they are bluffing but actually have a strong hand, or convince someone that they are pretending to bluff, but actually really are bluffing, and so on.

A cynic would say that life is poker writ large. We compete for limited resources, and one person's gain is another's loss. We are in a battle to the finish, where it is not physical strength that matters but the ability to connive, trick, and outplay. This makes sense from an evolutionary point of view. Traits emerge in the course of evolution only if they lead to enhanced reproductive success—better odds of surviving, more offspring. And "success" is a relative notion; it is not how well an animal does in an absolute sense that determines the fate of its genes; it is how well it does relative to everyone else. Natural selection is like the story of the two hikers who see a bear charging at them from a distance. One of them starts frantically putting on his running shoes. His friend shouts at him that it is useless; you can't outrun a bear. And the first guy shouts back: "I don't have to outrun the bear. I just have to outrun you."

But there is more to evolution than this straightforward competition between individuals. From an evolutionary perspective, our fates are yoked to those who share our genes: our kin, and most especially our children. In addition, many animals, including humans, have evolved to cooperate within a larger social setting than just the family; they can work together for mutual gain.

Because of this, our understanding of other minds shows itself in gentler ways. We can teach, an act that requires an exquisite appreciation of the mental states of those who know less than we do, along with the ability to craft our words and acts so as to foster in our pupils new mental and physical capacities. We can relate to others when working toward a common goal. This might mean something as simple as directing someone's attention by pointing and grunting, or as complex as engaging in negotiations with multiple participants. Our social nature also gives rise to the capacity for feelings such as empathy, compassion, and love.

In this chapter I will discuss human beings' understanding of one another in some detail, looking especially at how it develops in young children. Discoveries from developmental psychology, clinical research, and neuroscience provide the basis for the argument that runs through this book: some of our most interesting mental traits are best understood as unexpected by-products of our evolved capacity to understand and respond to the minds of other people.

But this is only half the story. We also have the evolved capacity to perceive and reason about material objects. If you place a rock on the ground, turn away for an instant, and then look back, you expect the rock to be where it was before. It should not hop away, dematerialize, or change into a camel. If you lean against a tree, you expect it to support your weight. If you grab the handle of a cup and pull, you expect the whole cup to move in the direction you are pulling; it should not stretch like rubber, turn to dust, or pull back from your grasp.

If these expectations are not met, you would suspect some sort of trickery, such as trapdoors or hidden wires. If everything were to go wrong at once—the cup pulls away from you, turns rubbery, and then disappears—you would feel as though you had been trapped in a painting by Salvador Dali.

These basic assumptions about how the physical world works are so entrenched and unconscious that it takes some effort to articulate them. Indeed, one of the main goals of psychology and philosophy is to define our most basic assumptions, to make explicit our naïve metaphysics, our understanding of the fundamental nature of reality. The developmental psychologist Elizabeth Spelke lists four properties that all humans assume physical objects possess:

1. *Cohesion*. Objects are connected masses of stuff that move as a whole. If you want to know where the boundaries of an object are, an easy test is to grab some portion of stuff and *pull*—what comes with what you are pulling belongs to the same object; what remains does not.

2. *Solidity*. Objects are not easily permeable by other objects; if you tap at an object with your finger, your finger does not penetrate.

3. *Continuity*. Objects move in continuous paths; they travel through space without gaps. An object would violate this rule if it disappeared from one location and reappeared in another.

4. *Contact*. Objects move through contact. A ball on a pool table is not going to move unless something contacts it; it will not run from the cue or come when it is called. The exceptions to this rule are animate creatures, like people and dogs, and also certain complex artifacts, such as robots and cars.

These assumptions we make about objects account for how we can understand and manipulate the external world. Yet they are unconscious. Therefore, it is possible for our conscious beliefs to clash with these instinctive assumptions. The philosopher George Berkeley held that we do not really perceive solid objects, because no such things exist. Some mystics believe that everything we experience is a dream. Some philosophers maintain that the idea of an enduring physical world is, at best, "a useful fiction." And many people take the lessons of modern physics as showing that, in reality, there exist only clouds of tiny particles, superstrings, or quanta.

I will return to these beliefs at the very end of this book. The point I wish to make here is that these skeptical positions, however sincere, are the products of conscious reasoning and deliberation, as distinct from the gut feelings that we all naturally possess.

PERFECT IDIOTS?

In December 2000 a front-page newspaper story described the results of a longitudinal study carried out by UCLA's Institute for Child Development in which a battery of intelligence tests was administered to over 3,500 babies. The babies were tested on tasks such as escaping from a room filled with cyanide gas, getting to shore after being left in the center of Lake Erie with only a nautical map for navigation, and preparing a meal with simple tools such as a can opener. Without exception, the babies failed to escape from the room, read the map, or prepare a meal. When placed in a torrential downpour, chickens, dogs, and worms were able to seek shelter, but the human babies were not. The scientists concluded, "Human babies, long thought by psychologists to be highly inquisitive and adaptable, are actually extraordinarily stupid."

The story was actually from the satirical newspaper *The Onion,* and the target of the satire was the babies-are-smart research discussed in the popular press. But the conclusion reached would have made perfect sense throughout much of intellectual history. William James famously described the mental life of a baby as "a blooming buzzing confusion," and in 1762, the French philosopher Jean-Jacques Rousseau made this point in harsher terms:

> We are born capable of learning, knowing nothing, perceiving nothing. Suppose a child born with the size and strength of manhood, entering upon life full grown like Pallas from the brain of Jupiter, such a child-man would be a perfect idiot, an automaton, a statue without motion and almost without feeling; he would see and hear

nothing, he would recognize no one, he could not turn his eyes towards what he wanted to see.

This conviction that newborns have no mental abilities whatsoever used to be the mainstream view in developmental psychology, and there was good reason to take it seriously. For instance, the Swiss psychologist Jean Piaget, who founded the modern study of child development, observed that if you take an attractive toy and put it in front of an eight-month-old, the baby will grab at it. But if you then cover the toy with a cloth—right while the baby is looking at it!—the baby acts as if the toy were no longer there. Babies make no attempt to lift the cloth to retrieve it, even though they are easily capable of this physical act. This discovery has been replicated over and over again; if you have access to a small baby, you can see it for yourself.

Piaget concluded that babies lack a sense of "object permanence"—they have no understanding that objects persist over time. Out of sight, out of mind. This fit in nicely with the account of philosophers such as Berkeley, who suggested that object understanding emerges only once babies begin to purposefully move through space and manipulate objects. These philosophers reasoned that because visual experience is only two-dimensional—the light that hits our eyes is akin to patterns of paint splashing onto two canvases—touch is necessary for us to understand that we live in a three-dimensional world.

According to an opposing intellectual tradition, considerable understanding is indeed required to appreciate the world of objects, but this understanding does not come from experience. Rationalist philosophers such as Plato, Descartes, and Kant have argued that much of our understanding of the physical world transcends our experience; we are born with it.

What then about the incompetence of babies? Psychologists have long appreciated that knowledge can surpass behavior; what one knows is very different from how one acts. This is particularly so for babies, who have problems planning coordinated physical action. Perhaps they are smarter than they look.

It is difficult to learn about the mental life of any creature that cannot use language, but a baby poses special challenges. Mature nonhumans, although nonverbal, are physically adroit. Chimpanzees can easily express their preferences through coordinated action; pigeons peck; rats run mazes; and so on. But young babies just lie there, crying or gurgling. (Just *try* to get a six-month-old to run a maze.) In addition, ethical issues arise with studies of humans of any age. One standard way to test animals is to starve them to 80 percent of their normal body weight and then reward their performance on complex tasks by giving them food. Parents are understandably unwilling to let us do this with their babies.

One might imagine that we can learn about what babies understand by scanning their brains in some way, using modern techniques of neuroscience. So far, however, these techniques remain crude and often cannot be done with babies because they are too dangerous, or because they require that the subject remain awake but very still for a long period of time. In any event, the main problem with such methods is that the data they provide—on the brain's electrical activity, blood flow, and oxygen use—do not tell us much about the specifics of mental life. Even for adults, it is unusual for the techniques of neuroscience to provide insights that we had not already obtained through simpler means.

Fortunately, we do not have to wait for neuroscience. Babies may have little control over their bodies, but they can willingly move their heads and eyes. And what a baby looks at can tell you something about how it sees the world. This is because babies are like adults in some regards. If they see the same thing over and over again, they get bored and look away. If they see something new or unexpected, they look longer. Thus, analyzing looking time can tell us what babies think of as being "the same thing" and what they see as being "new or unexpected."

Imagine a wide barrier. From behind the barrier a stick pokes out from the top and another stick pokes out from below, and the two parts move back and forth in tandem, as shown in figure 1.1.

An adult looking at this image will assume that it is of a single stick with its middle obscured. Do babies make the same assumption? The way to tell is to let them look at this image, then take away the barrier and show them either one stick or two sticks. The psychologists Philip Kellman and Elizabeth Spelke found that three-month-olds look longer when the barrier is removed and the two stick parts are unconnected than they do when the barrier is removed and they see just a single stick. Looking longer at the two sticks indicates surprise, so we can infer that the babies expected to see just one stick. Contrary to Piaget, then, babies are not entirely reliant on their senses for information; they sometimes have expectations about parts of objects that are out of sight. A similar study done with newborn chicks obtained the same result.

What about when a baby sees an object and then the entire object is hidden from view? Consider now the following study, done by my colleague Karen Wynn. You see an empty stage. A hand places a single Mickey Mouse doll on the stage. A screen is placed in front of the doll to hide it from view. Then the hand brings out another Mickey Mouse doll and places it out of sight behind the screen. Then the screen is removed. As an adult, you know that one Mickey plus another Mickey equals two Mickeys, so there should be two, not one or three.

Wynn finds that five-month-olds have the same expectation. They can keep a running count of how many Mickeys exist behind a screen, showing that they know full well that objects persist when they are out of sight. When this was reported in 1992, it caused quite a stir—*Can babies really add and subtract?* In fact it is a remarkably

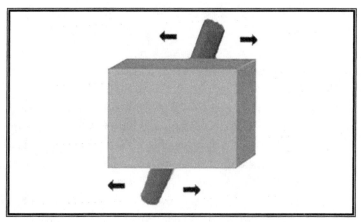

Figure 1.1 One stick or two?

robust finding, and has been replicated in several laboratories. The experiment has never been done with baby chicks, but has been done with different types of nonhuman primates, including macaques and tamarins, and also with pet dogs, and these studies all find that the animals understand object permanence.

Other studies have explored the four object principles discussed earlier:

1. Cohesion: If a hand pulls at an object, babies expect the entire object to go with the hand; if it comes off in pieces, they are surprised, showing an expectation that objects are *cohesive*.

2. Continuity: Imagine a stage with two vertical barriers separated in space. A small object, like a box, goes behind the barrier on the left, continues between the barriers, goes behind the barrier on the right, and comes out the other side. Adults see this is a single object, and so do babies. Now imagine that a box goes behind the barrier on the

left, there is a pause, and then a box emerges from the
screen on the right, never appearing in the gap. Adults assume that there are two boxes here, not one. Babies make
the same assumption; they expect *continuity*.

3. Solidity: If an object is put immediately behind a screen,
   and then the screen tilts backward, babies expect it to
   stop moving—it should hit the object. When it goes
   through the space that should be occupied by the hidden
   object (a trapdoor is used), babies look longer. They expect objects to be *solid*.

4. Contact: One object heads toward another, but the second
   object moves away an instant before the first object hits it.
   For babies, just as with adults, this action-at-a-distance is
   surprising; it violates the expectation of *contact*—that objects can only influence each other by touching.

There are limits to what babies know about the behavior of objects. In one study, babies are shown an empty stage. A screen rises
up to hide the center of the stage, there is a pause, then the screen
drops . . . to reveal a box. Adults see this as a trick, the laboratory
equivalent of a rabbit out of a hat. Babies, on the other hand, are
bored; they see nothing unusual here. For reasons that are not entirely clear, the understanding that objects do not blink *into* existence is a fairly late developmental accomplishment, which is in
sharp contrast to the natural understanding that objects do not
blink *out of* existence.

Another example comes from the work of the psychologist Renée
Baillargeon and her colleagues, who carried out several studies looking at babies' understanding of when things fall. For each of the
three pictures shown in figure 1.2, adults think that the black object
is not fully supported and should fall. But this understanding comes
in stages. Three-month-olds, the youngest children tested, share the

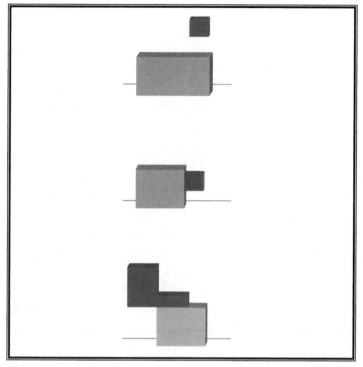

Figure 1.2 Violations of gravity.

adult intuitions about the scene depicted in the top picture: they think that the box should fall, and so when it hangs in midair they look longer. Only babies who are about five months old look longer at the display in the middle panel, and only children past their first birthday think there is anything weird about the bottom one.

These results show that although babies enter the world with a foundational understanding of what objects are and how they act, it is incomplete, and this foundation grows. Some of this improvement might be due to maturation of the brain—like the rest of the body, the brain changes rapidly in the early years of life, and this might cause corresponding increases in knowledge. But some of the improvement is plainly due to experience. In fact, cognitive psychologists have discovered that even some otherwise savvy adults can be confused about the behavior of objects. Here is a classic example.

What path does a ball take when it shoots out of a C-shaped tube?

Just under half of the adults tested say that it continues moving in a curving path. If this was your answer, you are in good company; it was Aristotle's understanding of motion as well. But, as Newton could have told you, it is not correct. The ball has no memory, and so once it pops out of the tube it will move in a straight line. People get this wrong because ball-popping-out-of-curved-tube is an unusual event, one that does not correspond to intuitively basic principles.

If lack of experience is to blame for the tube mistake, then adults should do a lot better when given a similar problem but in a domain that they are more familiar with:

What path does water take when it shoots out of a C-shaped hose?

This is a lot easier: nobody thinks that the water continues to curve. Apparently, natural selection equips humans—and other animals—with a foundational understanding of what objects are and how they behave. But the rest of the understanding of the physical world awaits the lessons of experience.

THE SOCIAL BABY

Even very young babies treat people differently from objects. If babies see a moving object become motionless, they lose interest. But if they interact with a person, and then the person's face becomes still and stays that way, they get upset. (You would too.) Babies expect faces not only to move, but to move in ways that are appropriate responses to their own actions. In one study, two-month-olds were seated across from a TV screen displaying their mother. When the mother interacts with the babies by means of real-time video-conferencing, babies enjoy it. But if there is a time delay of a few seconds, babies freak out; they turn away from the screen and get upset.

Babies prefer to look at faces more than just about anything else, and they have a special preference for the faces they are most familiar with—usually their moms'. They can distinguish happy faces from sad faces. And they imitate faces; the psychologist Andrew Meltzoff discovered that even newborns respond to the expression of an experimenter: when the experimenter sticks out his tongue, the babies tend to razz him back. This is very impressive. These babies have never looked in a mirror, so they have to know instinctively that the tongue they are looking at corresponds to that thing in their own mouth that they have never seen before.

Babies also have expectations about hands. Imagine a display with two different objects and a hand reaches for one of them. Babies expect that if the objects switch locations, the hand should change locations too and continue to pursue the same object. (This expectation is special to hands; one gets a different result if it is a stick that pokes at the object.) Hands are attached to people, and people have goals, and babies seem to understand that a reasonable goal for a person is to reach for a particular object, not to go to a specific location.

As they get older, babies start to show off these abilities in the real world. Before their first birthday, they are sensitive to where an adult is looking at or pointing to, and can use this information to figure out what he or she is paying attention to. They can attend to the emotions of others; if babies are crawling toward an area that might be dangerous and an adult makes a horrified or disgusted face, babies know enough to stay away. And they can do their own pointing, showing, and requesting. For instance, a baby who cannot yet talk can get someone to hand over an interesting object by waving toward it and grunting. By their first birthday, babies are social beings.

As best we know, there is nothing special about our species when it comes to knowledge of the physical world. Whenever there has been a careful comparison, it turns out that the same understanding of objects that you find with human babies shows up in other animals, particularly other primates. They seem to think about bodies the same way that we do.

But the situation is very different with regard to social understanding. Take something as seemingly simple as pointing. As I just mentioned, babies come to appreciate that adults make pointing gestures to establish their focus of interest, and babies are soon able to make these gestures themselves. This might seem like an easy thing to learn, but it involves a kind of mindreading—a recognition that people attend to some things and not others. Chimpanzees, our closest evolutionary relative, are much smarter than human babies in many regards, but not in this one. In the wild, they do not show, offer, or point to objects, despite the clear adaptive advantages of being able to do so. There have been efforts to teach chimps to point in order to get food, but these have met with limited success.

A host of other studies reveal that nonhuman animals have problems with related tasks that young children find fairly simple, such as inferring what someone knows about from the direction in which they are looking. Nobody would deny that chimpanzees and other primates have *some* social understanding, particularly with regard to day-to-day dealings with their kin and allies. But these findings suggest that the human capacity for mindreading might be qualitatively different from that of any other species. (Interestingly, recent studies suggest that *dogs* outperform chimps on many tasks involving social reasoning, presumably because dogs hunt in packs and also possibly because these capacities have been carefully bred into them by humans.)

If anything, people are overly eager to attribute mental states. In 1944, the social psychologists Fritz Heider and Mary-Ann Simmel made a simple movie in which geometrical figures—circles, squares, triangles—moved in certain systematic ways that were designed to tell a certain tale. When shown this movie, people instinctively described the figures as if they were specific people (bullies, victims, heroes) with goals and desires, and they repeated back pretty much the same story that the psychologists had intended to tell. Further research has established that you do not even need to use bounded figures; you can get much the same effect with moving dots and even with moving groups such as swarms of tiny squares. Animators have long been able to exploit this tendency when they create films in which inanimate objects come to life, like the mop and pail that conspire against Mickey Mouse in Walt Disney's *Fantasia*.

The same tendency to ascribe intention to inanimate objects manifests itself in less contrived circumstances, a phenomenon known as anthropomorphism. In his book *Faces in the Clouds,* the anthropologist Stewart Guthrie presents anecdotes and experiments showing that people will sometimes perceive the following things as having human characteristics: airplanes, automobiles, bags, bells, bicycles, boats, bottles, buildings, cities, clouds, clothing, earthquakes, fire, fog, food, garbage, hats, hurricanes, insects, locks, leaves, the moon, mountains, paper, pens, plants, pottery, rain, the sun, rivers, rocks, sirens, swords, tools, toys, trains, trees, volcanoes, water, and wind. We are so hypersensitive to signs of agency that we see intention where all that really exists is artifice or accident. As Guthrie puts it: the clothes have no emperor.

Babies are similarly trigger-happy. When babies see a film of patterns of lights that move in a human-looking fashion (because people with bright lights on their shoulders, elbows, hips, and knees were filmed moving around in darkness), they look at them longer than at moving light patterns that do not have a human source. Babies also prefer to look at circles that appear to be chasing each other than at two independently moving circles.

How can researchers be sure that babies see moving objects not only as alive but as having mental states? Maybe babies are just responding to the animacy of these displays, and make no assumptions about the presence of a mind behind the movements. But some recent studies do suggest that they treat animated objects as beings with psychological states. When 12-month-olds see one object chasing another, they seem to understand that it really is *chasing*, acting with the goal of catching someone else—they expect it to continue its pursuit along the most direct path, and are surprised when it does otherwise.

A more complex attribution shows up in a study I did in collaboration with Valerie Kuhlmeier and Karen Wynn. We showed babies a movie in which a circle tries to get up a hill. On some occasions, a triangle would gently push the circle from the bottom, apparently helping it up; on other occasions, a square would push it down from the top, seeming to thwart its desire. This is how adults perceive the movie. Do babies see this in the same way?

We tested babies' assumptions by later showing them movies where the circle sits between the triangle and the square, and then either approaches the triangle or the square. Twelve-month-olds, but not younger children, seem to expect the ball to approach the one that helped it and avoid the one that hindered it. My own interpretation of this behavior—admittedly a bit exuberant—is that the 12-month-olds assume that the circle *likes* the triangle and *hates* the square.

Mindreading abilities develop considerably in the second year of life. In a particularly clever study, children were shown two bowls, one of goldfish crackers and one containing broccoli. The experimenter would look cheerfully at the broccoli and say "Yum!" and make a disgusted face toward the crackers and say "Yuck!" Then the experimenter would hold out her hand and ask, "Can you give me some?" implicitly asking for the food she has expressed a liking for. Fourteen-month-old babies fail at the task of giving the experimenter what she wants and give her the food that *they* prefer—inevitably the crackers. But 18-month-olds succeed in giving the experimenter the one that she showed a preference for, broccoli, even though it is not their own choice. This shows that children before their second birthday not only understand that people have desires, they also know that others' desires might differ from their own.

BAD AT POKER

Once they start to speak, children show their knowledge of their own and other people's minds in a more direct way. They talk about mental states. The psychologists Karen Bartsch and Henry Wellman collected some nice examples of this. Here is a simple illustration that a two-year-old named Eve knows something about her own mental processes:

Adult: Would you like to have a cookie?
Eve: I want some cookie. Cookies, that make me happy.

A three-year-old named Abe seems to appreciate that other people can have views about the world that conflict with his own:

Abe: Some people don't like hawks. They think they have. . . they are slimy.
Mother: What do you think?
Abe: I think they are good animals.

My favorite is this one, also from a three-year-old, who explicitly recognizes that his mental state now is different from his mental state in the past. Prior to this exchange he had been eating glue.

Adam: I don't like it.
Adult: Why would you put that in your mouth?
Adam: I thought it was good.

Despite these impressive abilities, developmental psychologists have noted certain striking limitations on the part of babies and children. The most studied example of this is children's understanding of false beliefs. Consider the following problem:

Sally and Ann are together in a room that contains a basket and a box. Sally places her marble inside a basket, and leaves the room. While she is gone, naughty Ann moves her marble to the box. Sally returns. Where will Sally look for her marble?

This sort of "false-belief task" was first thought up by the philosopher Daniel Dennett in order to figure out how one can tell whether chimpanzees can reason about another actor's mental state. It is a good test for this purpose. To get to the right answer, you need to appreciate that Sally's action will be based not on how the world actually is but on how Sally *thinks* the world is; you need to take into account her mental state.

Four-year-olds typically pass this test, but younger children typically do not. They answer that Sally will look in the box, where the marble actually is. Their failure is consistent with more general observations that children of this age have a difficult time dealing with others' false beliefs. Three-year-olds are comically bad liars, the sorts who deny having eaten the cookies despite chocolate smeared on their face. (A friend of mine tells the story of how his family was going to surprise him on his birthday with a pie, and his three-year-old niece, who had repeatedly been told to keep this secret, walked up to him and shrieked, "There is no pie!") They are inept at hide-and-seek, because hiding requires a tacit appreciation that others' mental state will clash with how the world actually is—you are under the bed, but the seeker does not know you are under the bed. Three-year-olds always hide in the same place, or they tell you where they are going to hide, or insist that you hide in a certain location. They still enjoy the game, but their pleasure is not in fooling you, but in the theater—the parent's exaggerated pantomime of search, screaming with delight when they are found, and so on.

There is a lot of debate over why children have problems handling false-belief situations. One influential proposal is that children younger than four have a qualitatively different understanding of minds than adults do. Another possibility is that children have problems reasoning about false belief just because this sort of reasoning is *hard*, even for adults. And what is hard for adults is often impossible for young children.

Several factors make it hard. First, to succeed at a false-belief task, you have to hold in your mind two conflicting pictures of the world—the world as it really is (the marble is in the box) and the world as it is in someone's mind (the marble is in the basket). This double bookkeeping is difficult for two- and three-year-olds even in cases where the representations have nothing to do with beliefs. It sometimes poses problems for adults too, which is why some of us find it hard to lie: when you tell the truth, you simply have to consult what you know; when you lie, you have the extra job of keeping track of the alternative universe that you are constructing in another person's mind.

The psychologist Susan Birch explored a second source of difficulty. She has done a series of studies suggesting that children's failure at the false-belief task is partially because they suffer from an exaggerated version of a bias that adults possess, sometimes called *the curse of knowledge*: a pervasive assumption that others have the same knowledge that they do. Several studies have demonstrated that once someone knows something—such as the answer to a question, the value of a company, or whether someone is lying—he or she will tend to assume that others have the same knowledge. (This is one reason why teaching is so difficult.) And so the question of where Sally will look for the marble poses a challenge in part because the child has to understand that her own knowledge is not shared by Sally. Similarly, people tend to exaggerate the extent to which everyone shares their own desires. The failure of 14-month-olds in the broccoli/crackers task should come as no surprise to anyone who has non-standard tastes and has had to defend them against incredulous others ("How could you *not* like cheese/the Rolling Stones/heterosexual intercourse?").

Adults do generally manage to overcome the curse-of-knowledge. We can teach, and lie, and understand that Sally thinks the marble is in the basket even though we know it is in the box; and we come to grips with the vexing fact that others' tastes in food, music, and sex might be radically different from our own. It would be a mistake to assume that once children can succeed at the false-belief task (roughly at the age of four), they have the same mindreading powers that adults possess. Instead there is a gradual growth in the ability to reason about others' mental states. A seven-year-old might be able to pass the false-belief test and do a reasonable job of lying, but still stumble when exposed to situations that require complex attribution of mental states and assessments of others' knowledge, as when following the plot of a play such as *Hamlet* or a movie such as *The Sting*.

Even adults differ in the extent to which they choose to focus on mental states. In an old cartoon, two psychoanalysts pass each other in a conference. One says, "Hello," and the other thinks, "I wonder what he meant by *that*." There are also differences in the ability to mindread. Some of this might be inborn, but practice surely helps—the winners of the World Series of Poker got to be so good at figuring out what other players are thinking in large part because they have spent thousands of hours at the card table.

Practice is not the only thing that distinguishes adults from children. There is also knowledge, the specific knowledge that people acquire in different cultural settings. While objects are solid wherever you go, people—and people's minds—differ substantially across time and space. The sorts of beliefs and desires in the head of a shoemaker in medieval France differ in interesting ways from those of a member of a hunter-gatherer tribe in Papua New Guinea ten thousand years ago or of a modern-day reader of this book. Children have to learn the unique properties of people's minds within the culture in which they are raised. Since they are not born knowing which culture they will live in, some degree of learning is essential.

Superficial examples of this knowledge are the sorts of facts that one reads in guidebooks—these people are offended if you point your bare feet at them, those people will be surprised to encounter someone traveling without her family and will pity her, the natives in this culture will ridicule someone who does not drink alcohol or eat meat. These are crude attempts to summarize truths about a society that are known by its members.

This learning goes on throughout development. Most five-year-olds do not know that you can better remember a string of numbers by repeating them over and over again in your head, or that lack of food makes people grumpy. In many cultures, some information about people is purposefully kept from children. Indeed, the cultural critic Neil Postman has argued that one of the defining features of "childhood" as a social institution is that children are forbidden to know certain things about the world, the most obvious off-limits topic being adult sexuality.

You can see this ignorance in all sorts of ways. Children are notorious for acting in ways that would be considered inexcusably rude in an adult. They will often remark loudly on the physical features of people who look unusual ("Look, a fat lady!"). They are candid when receiving gifts that they do not like ("I already have one of these!"), and will discuss toilet matters openly ("I have to poop!"). None of this behavior is malicious. It is just that children do not know enough about what offends people.

Just like the child's understanding of physical bodies, the understanding of people's minds builds on a foundation that is already present. While children do need to learn about the *contents* of minds—what people typically believe, what makes them angry, and so on—they do not have to learn that other people know things and want things and have beliefs, emotions, desires, and feelings. This comes for free.

MINDBLINDNESS

How important is our understanding of people and objects to our existence? One way to answer this is to see what happens when adults or children lack this understanding. Also, by looking at what can go wrong in exceptional cases, we can learn how things work in the normal course of affairs.

Disorders in dealing with the physical world are typically the results of problems with perception (usually visual perception) and attention. For instance, in the disorder called "neglect," a person might be conscious only of what is on the right side of the visual world. Balint syndrome is an extreme version of neglect: those afflicted with this disorder can focus on only one object at a time, and the attention needs to be conscious. This can make them effectively blind: they walk into things, and they don't turn to people who approach. But if an experimenter places an object in front of them, they can see it perfectly clearly—so long as nothing else is there to steal away their limited attention.

There is no such thing, however, as a deficit that blots out object understanding, leaving its victim unable to appreciate that objects are cohesive and solid, travel in continuous paths, and move only through contact. That is, there is nothing similar in the world of bodies to the disorders that we find in the domains of social understanding.

In 1988, Dustin Hoffman won an Academy Award for his portrayal of an autistic man in the movie *Rain Man*. The character he played was socially bizarre and highly obsessional, and he possessed extraordinary mathematical powers. Hoffman provided a moving, and accurate, picture of what autism can be like, but it would be a mistake to take this as typical.

Indeed, the pendulum has swung with regard to how we think about autism. Oliver Sacks points out that the typical image used to be of "a profoundly disabled child, with stereotyped movements, perhaps head-banging, rudimentary language, almost inaccessible: a creature for whom very little future lies in store." In reality, some people with autism are very much like Hoffman's character; some are far more high-functioning and can live independently, such as Temple Grandin, a university professor who writes and lectures about her own experience with autism. Sadly, others fit Sacks's description, and spend their days rocking back and forth, silent and withdrawn.

Autism occurs in roughly one out of every 1,000 babies, and most often strikes boys. Its dominant feature is a lack of social connectedness—autistic children typically show impairments in communication (about a third do not speak at all), in imagination (they do not tend to engage in imaginative play), and, most of all, in the ability to interact appropriately with others. Their socialization is impaired. They do not seem to enjoy the company of others, they don't hug, they are hard to reach out to. It is often said that autistic children are particularly good-looking—when the psychiatrist Leo Kanner first described the disorder in 1943, he listed an alert and attractive appearance as one of its features. Certainly autistic children don't look in any way unusual or retarded; there is often an impression of an aloof intelligence. (My brother Howard is autistic, and he is quite handsome and looks like a perfectly normal man, but if you were to approach him to start a conversation, he would turn away from you; he does not speak.)

This lack of sociability, when combined with other features of autism, including obsession with routine, bizarre fixations, and occasionally dangerous behavior such as head-banging and violent tantrums, makes it difficult for parents to raise these children. The author Nick Hornby, the father of an autistic child, expresses his frustration when he asks, "How do you reach those who, for the most part, have no language, and no particular compulsion to acquire it, who are born without the need to explore the world, who would rather spin round and round in a circle, or do the same jigsaw over and over again, than play games with their peers, who won't make eye contact, or copy, and fight bitterly (and sometimes literally, with nails and teeth and small fists) for the right to remain sealed in their own world?"

We do not know very much about autism and autistic people. We do not know precisely what is wrong with their brains. We do not know how to explain certain puzzling symptoms that are not obviously related to their social deficit, such as an obsession with routine or a hypersensitivity to certain sounds. We do not even know whether autism is a single disorder that varies in severity, or many disorders. Some investigators have proposed that certain high-functioning individuals should be seen as having a different deficit altogether (Asperger Syndrome), as opposed to suffering from a mild form of autism.

We do know that autism is not the product of savage treatment by parents. If that were true, then children who clearly have been abused would tend to be autistic (they are not), and the siblings of autistic children, who would presumably have experienced much the same brutality, should also tend to be autistic (they are not). Nevertheless, in the not-so-distant past, psychologists such as Bruno Bettelheim convinced many people that the cause of autism was a cold maternal figure—the dreaded "refrigerator mother"—and mothers of children with autism were sent off for psychoanalysis to try to determine precisely why they were such terrible parents.

The damage done to these families is hard to imagine, and should give pause to certain contemporary psychologists eager to attribute, with little supporting evidence, all sorts of bad traits—from conduct disorder to bedwetting—to the sins of the mothers. We know now that autism emerges very early in development, that it is not caused by any sort of parental abuse (though it may be related to some sort of trauma prior to birth), and that it has a strong genetic basis. The psychologists Alison Gopnik, Andrew Meltzoff, and Patricia Kuhl nicely summarize it this way: "The senselessly cruel mother here is Mother Nature."

To make sense of autism, we have to go beyond listing the symptoms and ask what is different about some people's minds that gives rise to these symptoms. The psychologists Simon Baron-Cohen, Uta Frith, and Alan Leslie propose that individuals with autism suffer from "mindblindness." In the most extreme form, people are seen as nothing more than objects—objects that move in unpredictable ways and make unexpected noises, and so are frightening things.

While Hornby tells us what it is like to try to teach an autistic child, Gopnik tells us what it is like to *be* an autistic child:

This is what it's like to sit round the dinner table. At the top of my field of vision is a blurry edge of nose, in front are waving hands. . . . Around me bags of skin are draped over chairs and stuffed into pieces of cloth, they shift and protrude in unexpected ways. . . . Two

dark spots near the top of them swivel relentlessly back and forth. A
hole beneath the spots fills with food and from it come a stream of
noises. Imagine that the noisy skin-bags suddenly moved toward you
and their noises grew loud, and you have no idea why, no way of explaining them or predicting what they would do next.

If this mindblindness theory is true, one could expect such
mindblind people to be poor at social reasoning tasks. They are.
One of the striking findings of studies of autism is that even high-
functioning autistic people have special problems with tasks involving an understanding of the mental states of others such as the
false-belief task described above.

They also have problems with the easier stuff. Normally developing children like to look at faces; autistic children do not. They do
not tend to point things out, or to show things to their parents, or
to engage in pretend play. When faced with an unfamiliar object,
normally developing children look at their mother or father and
look back at the object, using the adult's expression as a way to assess the properties of this strange thing. Typically, autistic children
do not do this. In one study, a small remote-controlled robot would
approach a three-year-old while the child's parent stood to the side
and pretended to be terrified, making fearful expressions and
sounds. The normally developing children kept away from the robot, but the autistic children ignored the parent's communications
and showed no fear at all.

There is some sign that the deficit of autism also extends to empathy. In a study with 20-month-olds, the experimenter and the
child would play a game with a toy hammer and a plastic object. At
one point the experimenter would act as if he had hit his thumb
with his hammer and would yelp with pain and stop the game.
None of the 10 autistic children studied showed any sign of concern, while most (but not all!) of the normally developing children

were plainly upset. This lack of appreciation of the pain of others fits with more casual observations. Oliver Sacks recounts the story of an intelligent 12-year-old autistic girl who approached a teacher and said of another student, "Joanie is making a funny noise." Joanie was weeping.

What can we make of people with autism who fare very well, such as Temple Grandin? It is likely that they have a less severe disorder to start with. But they are also capable of compensating for what they lack, using conscious effort and hard work to do what comes naturally to most everyone else. Temple Grandin calls herself an "anthropologist on Mars" and explains how she studies people's behavior as a complex and alien system that can only be worked out through explicit research, reviewing her interactions with people over and over in her mind so as to make sense of them.

Such high-functioning autistic people differ from the rest of us in intriguing ways. For instance, when shown animations of moving geometrical figures of the sort that normally developing children describe in intentional terms—the triangle is chasing the circle, the circle is frightened and tries to hide—the individuals with autism often describe them in a purely physical way: the triangle moves suddenly to the left, the circle drops down at a 45-degree angle, and so on.

In another study, both normal and autistic adults watched movie clips from Edward Albee's classic *Who's Afraid of Virginia Woolf?* A computer system scanned their eye movements to determine where they were looking for each fraction of a second. During a heated argument between the husband and wife (played by Richard Burton and Elizabeth Taylor), normal people looked intently at the characters' eyes, their own eyes darting back and forth to see how the characters were reacting. Autistic people looked at any source of motion, such as the characters' mouths, and sometimes at salient objects in the background. When they did look at faces, studies of their brain activity showed that the parts of the brain typically associated with faces were not responding; instead, the autistic brains responded to faces as if they were objects.

If problems with understanding the minds of others fall along a continuum, what would be the mildest deficit imaginable? According to the psychologist Simon Baron-Cohen, to be male is to have a very minor form of autism. Or, to put it in the more careful way that Baron-Cohen does, perhaps people with autism suffer from an extreme and exaggerated version of the typical male profile.

Something about this notion makes sense. Most people with autism are male. More than that, though, the sort of intense and socially awkward behavior that one finds in high-functioning individuals with autism looks a lot like the stereotype of a gawky male nerd. In general, Baron-Cohen argues, women are better at understanding minds than men are. They are more sensitive to the emotional states of others and also are better at reasoning about other people's beliefs and desires.

Some of the evidence for this sex difference is indirect. Universally, males tend to be more physically violent than females, more inclined toward roughhousing as children, and far more prone as adults to commit murder—what Baron-Cohen dryly describes as "the ultimate example of lack of empathy." Other evidence is more telling, and has to do with babies and young children.

- One-day-old baby girls look longer at a face than at a moving mechanical mobile; boys show the opposite preference.
- Little girls make more eye contact at age one than little boys do, and the amount of eye contact made by children at this age is predicted by the level of prenatal testosterone, a male sex hormone: the more testosterone, the less eye contact.

- As soon as children develop enough to show signs of empathy and caring, girls show it more than boys. One-year-old girls are more likely than boys to help others in distress.
- Girls consistently outperform boys at tasks, such as the false-belief task, that involve inferring what other people are thinking and are better at decoding facial expressions and nonverbal gestures.
- Boys are more likely than girls to suffer from disorders involving problems with mindreading and empathy, including autism, conduct disorder, and psychopathy.

We are dealing with averages here; there are plenty of empathetic and socially savvy men around, alongside plenty of coldhearted and nerdy women. And nobody denies that cultural factors of all sorts can exaggerate or inhibit these differences. But given that the foundations of mindreading are inborn, it is not entirely surprising to find differences in mindreading abilities tied to significant biological distinctions, such as that between males and females.

SURPLUS CAPACITY

None of what I have discussed so far is unexpected from the perspective of a biologist. Humans have evolved a foundational appreciation of the physical and social worlds. To see how adaptive this is, just consider what life is like for a person with Balint syndrome or severe autism, and imagine that person struggling to survive in the hunter-gatherer environment of our distant ancestors. There really is no mystery as to the origin of these adaptive capacities; the process of natural selection provides an excellent explanation for how such traits can evolve in a species.

The existence of these capacities is also perfectly consistent with current psychological theories of how the mind works. Psychologists agree that the brain contains processes, biases, and knowledge structures that underlie how we perceive and act in the world, and that some of these are specialized for certain domains or problems. (In an earlier time, these specializations would be called habits of the mind or faculties or instincts; now they are sometimes called modules or mental organs.) Although there is disagreement as to the extent of this specialization and how it emerges, its existence is not in question.

Now for the hard part. Humans have capacities that other creatures lack. Some of these, most notably language, may be biological adaptations in the standard Darwinian sense that they increase the chance of survival, but others plainly are not. It is likely that an understanding of physical bodies and social beings has evolved because those who possess this understanding have an increased shot at survival and reproduction; but it is a lot less clear that this can be said of other human features such as the capacity for religious belief, artistic practice, and moral thought.

One of Charles Darwin's contemporaries, Alfred Russell Wallace, who had independently discovered natural selection, made a related point; he argued that "higher" intellectual capacities could not have resulted from natural selection, because, he said, they only exist in certain societies. Some groups of humans ("savages") got along just fine without them. Wallace concluded that these capacities must have a divine origin: "[M]an's body may have developed from that of a lower animal form under the law of natural selection but. . . we possess intellectual and moral faculties which could not have been so developed but must have had another origin and for this origin we can only find an adequate cause in the unseen universe of Spirit."

This sentiment has been echoed more recently by John Polkinghorne, a mathematical physicist and Anglican priest, who is the recent winner of the million-dollar Templeton Prize for "research and discoveries about spiritual realities." Polkinghorne agrees that evolution would have shaped our minds so as to help us understand the world around us, because such an understanding helps us survive and reproduce. But biology cannot explain our uniquely human mental powers, what he describes as "our surplus intellectual capacity." Polkinghorne writes that "it beggars belief that this is simply a fortunate by-product of the struggle for life." In 1996 the pope made a similar claim when he conceded that evolution can explain the origin of animals and the bodies of humans but asserted that "the spiritual soul is immediately created by God." I would imagine that if Descartes were alive today, he would express much the same sentiment.

Darwin had no sympathy for Wallace's point of view and responded angrily, "I hope you have not murdered too completely your own and my child." In the margin of Wallace's book he wrote, "No!!" and underlined it twice. Darwin well understood that it is fully compatible with the process of natural selection that something can evolve for one purpose and later be turned to another purpose, either with or without subsequent modification, a process he called "preadaptation." Contemporary biologists have explored different variations of this theme, using the terms "exaptation" or "spandrels."

The general idea is simple enough: The nose, having evolved as a sense organ, can be used to support glasses; our feet, evolved for locomotion, can be used to kick a soccer ball. Furthermore, our brains can do things in this modern world that provide no obvious reproductive advantage. A mind that has evolved to respond with sexual arousal in situations with actual people (adaptive) can respond the same way to pornographic movies (nonadaptive); a preference for sweet fruit (adaptive) can drive one to gorge on candy (nonadaptive). This is one way we can explain the origin of nonadaptive, uniquely human, capacities: they are biological accidents.

But just to say that some mental capacity is a by-product of a biological adaptation falls short of an explanation. At best it is a clue to where an explanation can be found. One needs to be specific about the precise nature of the adaptation, and the way its existence leads to the capacity that one is interested in.

One particularly promising explanation for our uniquely human powers focuses on the transforming power of language. Some researchers suggest that once our species evolved language, our enhanced ability to communicate made our social and mental lives qualitatively richer than that of any other species. Furthermore, language allowed us to accumulate the insights of the past, originally in terms of memorized narratives and then through the written word. If a strange virus emerged and permanently stripped people of the ability to use and understand language—turned us all into aphasics, those unfortunate people rendered silent because of damage to their brains through stroke or injury—just about all of our science, technology, and culture would be obliterated within a generation. A stronger claim is that when children learn language it profoundly enhances their intellectual powers. It makes them *smarter*. Daniel Dennett presents an extreme version of this proposal when he writes, "Perhaps the kind of mind you get when you add language to it is so different from the kind of mind you can have without language that calling them both minds is a mistake."

In the rest of this book, I will explore a different sort of by-product theory. Without denying the role of language, I will suggest that some of the most interesting aspects of mental life are a consequence of the two capacities discussed in this chapter: our understanding of material bodies and our understanding of people. We see the world as containing bodies and souls, and this explains much of what makes us human.

PART II

THE MATERIAL REALM

2

ARTIFACTS

> Virtually all urban sensual experience has been touched by human hands, and thus the vast majority of us experience the physical world. . . as filtered through the process of design.
> —Henry Petroski, *The Evolution of Useful Things*

IT IS EMOTIONALLY draining to interact with autistic children. Unlike children with Down syndrome, who are affectionate and cuddly, many autistic children are not drawn to people. When Leo Kanner first described autism in 1943, he quoted the mother of a boy named Charles as saying, "What upsets me most is that I can't reach my baby. . . . He would pay no attention to me and show no recognition of me if I enter the room. The most impressive thing is his detachment and his inaccessibility."

It is sometimes said that such children treat people like objects. My experience is that this can be literally true. As a teenager I worked as a counselor in a camp for autistic children, and one afternoon, a severely impaired seven-year-old boy walked up to me and placed his hands on my shoulders. I was surprised, and touched, by what appeared to be a spontaneous act of affection. But then he tightened his grip, jumped up, pressed his feet on my legs, and started to climb. It turned out that I was standing next to a high shelf, and he was using me as a ladder so that he could get to an attractive toy.

Children with autism extend physical and mechanical modes of understanding to inappropriate entities, ones who, like me, are better understood in terms of mental states. (It would have been simpler if he had just asked me to get him the toy.) For the rest of us the opposite is true: we extend our capacity for mindreading into the object realm.

Sometimes this is reasonable. It makes sense to consider intention when dealing with artifacts such as sweaters, chairs, and clocks—people have actually made these things. But we go further than this. As a consequence of our evolved capacity for mindreading, even young children are prone to see much of the physical and biological world as existing for a purpose, consisting of artifacts created by a divine designer.

SPLITTERS AND LUMPERS

John Locke once imagined a language in which every individual object, not just individual people but also individual rocks, leaves, and clouds, had its own name. Three hundred years later, the Argentinean writer Jorge Luis Borges took this notion a step further and introduced a character, Funes the Memorious, with a perfect memory: "[H]e knew by heart the forms of the southern clouds at dawn on the 30th of April, 1882, and could compare them in his memory with the mottled streaks on a book in Spanish binding he had only seen once." Funes wanted a language capable of expressing his experiences and rejected Locke's proposal as too weak. For Funes, it would not be enough to name every individual. He wanted to have a distinct name for each experience with every individual. Now *this* would be a perfect language!

Or would it? Scientists distinguish between "splitters" and "lumpers," between those who favor fine-grained distinctions and those who tend to put entities together into broad categories. Funes is the most extreme splitter one can imagine, and there are times when such splitting, in thought and in language, is warranted. For example, we recognize that some entities, like children, deserve to be seen—and named—as distinct individuals.

For the most part, we are lumpers. Our minds have evolved to put things into categories and to ignore or downplay what makes these things distinct. Some categories are more obvious than others: all children understand the categories chairs and tigers; only scientists are comfortable with categories such as ungulates and quarks. (Genesis offers a particularly natural four-way distinction within the animate world: fish, fowl, beast, and man). What all categories share is that they capture a potential infinity of individuals under a single perspective. They lump.

Why does the mind work this way? Why don't we just store each instance as a precious and unique individual, like Funes did? One answer is that all of these discrete memories could not fit into our heads. Locke considered this at one point: "[I]t is beyond the power of human capacity to frame and retain distinct ideas of all the particular things we meet with: every bird and beast men saw; every tree and plant that affected the senses, could not find a place in the most capacious understanding." (For what it is worth, this is the boxer George Foreman's excuse for naming each of his five sons "George" and each of his five daughters "Georgetta"—he worried that his memory might fail and he would not be able to tell one child from another.) If we were to store in our memory a single distinct impression for each second of waking life, and never forget anything, we would die with billions of distinct memories.

The problem with this argument is that nobody knows whether or not a billion memories would exceed the capacity of human memory. We don't know whether a character such as Funes could really exist. And in any case, saving memory space is not a valuable goal in itself. If this were the whole problem, the mind would not need something as baroque as lumping—the simpler solution would be to just forget most of the individuals one encountered.

Locke eventually comes to a better answer: A perfect memory, one that treats each experience as a distinct thing-in-itself, is useless. The whole point of storing the past is to make sense of the present and to plan for the future. Without categories, everything is perfectly different from everything else, and nothing can be generalized or learned. There is no *savings*, no information gained. Borges was well aware of this, as he tells us that Funes sometimes would remember an entire day of his life, but it would take him an entire day to do so. (It is like the comedian Steven Wright's story of buying a map of the United States—actual size. He spent the summer folding it.)

We lump the world into categories so that we can learn. When we encounter something new, it is not entirely new; we know what to expect of it and how to act toward it. The psychologist Gregory Murphy begins *The Big Book of Concepts* with exactly this point:

> We seldom eat the same tomato twice, and we often encounter novel objects, people, and situations. Fortunately, even novel things are usually similar to things we already know, often exemplifying a category that we are familiar with. Although I've never seen this particular tomato before, it is probably like other tomatoes I have eaten and so is edible. . . . Concepts are a kind of mental glue, then, in that they tie our past experiences to our present interactions with the world.

Someone without the right concepts might well starve to death surrounded by tomatoes, "because he or she has never seen *those particular* tomatoes before and so doesn't know what to do with them." Without a concept "object" there would be no understanding of the physical world; without "person" and "friend" and "self" and "other," there would be no sense of the social world. Without concepts, we are helpless.

MORE THAN DULL CATALOGUES

Suppose someone ate her first tomato, found it satisfying, and concluded that other things that fell into the same category would be equally satisfying. But instead of grasping the category as including all and only tomatoes, instead she defined it like this:

Red things
or
Objects smaller than a gorilla
or
Things that are not televisions

This person would be in serious trouble as she attempted to chomp down on book covers, sweaters, and fire hydrants before ever zooming in on a tomato. If the purpose of placing things into categories is to make the right choices about how to act toward novel things, it is not enough to place them into categories; the categories have to be the right ones, like tomatoes or fruit, and not useless ones, like objects smaller than a gorilla.

What makes a category "the right one"? The answer is clear once we consider again what concepts are for. Tomato is a good category, because once you know something is a tomato, you know other things about it, including that it is good to eat. Once you know something is a chair, you know it is likely to support your weight; once you know something is a dog, you know it is likely to bark, eat meat, sleep, and so on. You know properties about these entities that are humanly relevant, and that distinguish them from other categories.

Such categories exist in the first place because objects are not randomly distributed in the universe with regard to the properties that they possess. Animals, for instance, fall into natural groups—such as species—because they are adapted to certain niches, and because the laws of genetics lead to resemblance within a category. Our minds have adapted to form categories that correspond to these natural discontinuities. As the paleontologist Stephen Jay Gould has pointed out, "Classifications are theories about the basis of natural order, not dull catalogues compiled only to avoid chaos."

With this is mind, we can go back to Borges and look at his fantastical report of how the Chinese encyclopedia *The Celestial Emporium of Benevolent Knowledge* divided the animal world into categories:

Those that belong to the Emperor
Embalmed ones
Those that are trained
Suckling pigs
Mermaids
Fabulous ones
Stray dogs
Those that are included in this classification
Those that tremble as if they were mad
Innumerable ones
Those drawn with a very fine camel's-hair brush
Others
Those that have just broken a flower vase
Those that resemble flies from a distance

This is a beautiful and clever list—as the writer Jennifer Ackerman puts it, "It rumples linear ideas of kind, blunts the sharp edge of category, and baffles hierarchy." But at the risk of being pedantic, I can now explain just what is so weird about many of these entries. Animals who have just broken a flower vase have nothing in common other than the fact that they have just broken a flower vase. Such a category is unnatural because it is trivial.

I can't resist adding that the same sort of rumpling, blunting, and baffling *can* be found in other classification schemes. Consider the different ways in which one can die.

Aged
Bleeding
Executed
Found dead in the streets
Grief
Killed by several accidents
Lethargy
Mother
Plague
Poisoned
Suddenly
Vomiting
Wolf

This list looks like a bad Borges imitation but it is genuine, taken from a "Table of casualties" in Britain in 1650. Bureaucracies can invent ways of sorting the world that differ sharply from those arising from science or common sense.

Once we understand the difference between a useful and useless category, we still need a theory of how our minds lock on to the useful ones. An omniscient God can see the world and intuitively know the relevant categories, but mortal beings cannot. We need to use, directly and inferentially, information that comes to us through our senses.

Take the categorization of animals. Given the task of establishing species boundaries, you could do pretty well just by using your eyes. If you cannot tell two creatures apart, it is reasonable to assume that they belong to the same species; if they are radically dissimilar—a worm and an eagle, say—you'd be wise to assume that they fall into different categories. Someone entirely innocent of the discoveries of science could, just by looking, produce a rough approximation to the world as seen by a biologist. Appearance is a useful beginning.

But to stop here would be to miss what is perhaps most important about how we make sense of the world. There is a crucial difference between what things look like and what they really are. Most of the creatures in nature have no grasp of this distinction. A frog is sensitive to flies and uses their patterns of motion to identify them, but the frog's brain has no way of entertaining the notion that something might move like a fly but not actually be a fly. Humans are smarter than frogs; we know that looking like a fly and being a fly are not one and the same.

Admittedly, people are often suckered by illusions, forgeries, frauds, and counterfeits. Indeed, even when we know full well that we are not dealing with the real thing, as when watching television, our minds can treat an image as real and generate responses such as hunger, fear, and disgust. This is particularly true of children, who have long had a deserved reputation for responding to the exterior qualities of things and not delving deeper.

Nevertheless, we can recognize genuine categories. We know that all that glitters is not gold; the plots of *Madame Butterfly* and *The Crying Game* do not bewilder us. Not our eyes but our deeper understanding of the world tells us that Chihuahuas and Great Danes belong to the same species, that marsupial mice share a category with kangaroos, or that a hummingbird, an ostrich, and a falcon are all birds but that a bat is not. Much of our mental life rests on an understanding that there are two ways to chop up the world, as it appears and as it really is. Hence most psychologists and philosophers have agreed that other considerations—such as patterns of language, cultural practices, and scientific discoveries—can sometimes override the way things appear to our senses.

It is sometimes surprising how much of our classification process is influenced by language and culture. Sue Hubbell gives an extreme example of this when she poses the question "How would we see an ape if we had not been told what it is?" What if it were not seen locked up in a zoo or on a nature channel? What if it had not been given a distinct label? Would we then know that it belonged to a different species from ours? When I first heard this question, my immediate response was that *of course* we would see an ape as distinct from a person. This would be obvious to any sane observer.

I was wrong. Some people upon first seeing nonhuman primates did not see them as separate species. The first Mediterranean people who came to Africa provided the following description of the inhabitants of an island:

> In the recess of this bay there was an island full of savage men. There were women, too, in even greater number. They had hairy bodies. . . . When we pursued them we were unable to take any of the men, for they all escaped, by climbing steep places and defending themselves with stones; but we took three of the women, who bit and scratched. . . and would not follow us. So we killed them and flayed them, and brought their skins to Carthage.

The natives had a name for this tribe of savage men and women: *Gorrilae.*

GET REAL

It is clear enough what we mean when we say that something looks like a tiger. But what do we mean when we say that something *is* a tiger? What makes such a claim true?

We have a particular way of thinking about objects whereby we ascribe to them a nature that transcends their appearance. This way of thinking was described by John Locke: "The real internal, but generally . . . unknown constitution of things, whereon their discoverable qualities depend, may be called their *essence*." Water, for instance, has certain observable properties—what it looks like, what it tastes like. But the chemical makeup of water, H_2O, is what makes it what it is.

Even when people do not know what the essences are, they believe that they exist. Long before anyone knew about the molecular structure of water, people understood that something might seem like water but not be water, or might not seem like water but actually be water; what makes something water has to do with hidden properties, not merely appearance.

Anthropologists often claim that a belief in the existence of essences—essentialism—is a product of Western culture, one that arose as the consequence of modern science. But many developmental psychologists have a different view, arguing that this essentialist mode of thought is actually a human universal, present even in young children. A considerable body of evidence supports this claim:

• Even nine-month-olds understand that objects of the same category share hidden properties. If they discover that a box produces a sound when you touch it in a certain way, they expect other boxes that look like it to produce the same sound. Older children will draw conclusions about shared properties even if the objects look different. In one set of studies, children three years old were shown a picture of an animal—say, a robin—and told that it had a hidden property, such as a certain chemical in its blood. Then they had to decide whether this property is shared with an animal that looks similar but belongs to a different category, such as a bat, or with an animal that looks different but belongs to the same category, such as a pelican. The three-year-olds chose correctly; for them, as for adults, sameness of category is more important than similarity of appearance.

• Like adults, children believe that if you remove the insides of a dog (its blood and bones), it is no longer really a dog and cannot do typical dog activities such as barking and eating dog food, whereas if you remove the outsides of a dog (its fur), it retains its most important doggy properties. And they are more willing to give a common name to objects described as sharing common internal properties ("the same sort of stuff inside") than superficial properties ("lives in the same kind of zoo and the same kind of cage"). In general, when thinking about and talking about categories, children give greater weight to internal hidden properties than observable external features.

• In the most dramatic set of studies, children were shown pictures of a series of transformations where animals were gradually modified in their appearance: a porcupine was surgically altered to resemble a cactus; a tiger was stuffed into a lion suit so that it looked like a lion; a real dog was modified to look like a toy. When the transformations were radical enough, children rejected them—they insisted that it was still a porcupine, a tiger, and a dog, regardless of what it looked like. In a child's mind, to be a specific animal is more than to have a certain appearance, it is to have a certain internal structure. It is only when the transformations are described as changing the *innards* of the animals—presumably, their essences—that children, like adults, take them as changing the type of animal itself.

Why do children believe in essences? It is not the result of formal education (these studies involved preschool children), nor is it likely to be learned from their parents (even highly educated parents in college towns rarely talk to their children about insides and essences,

and working-class parents do so even less.) Moreover, this essentialist bias appears to be universal. Although cross-cultural research
finds differences in the precise way that the essences are understood—where urban Americans might talk about genes, Yoruba
farmers might talk instead about "structure from heaven"—essentialism shows up in every society that has been studied. It appears to
be a basic component of how we think about the world.

This should not be surprising. Essentialism is an adaptive stance
to take toward the natural world. In biology, animals fall into
groups not merely because they look alike, but because of shared
evolutionary history. Appearance does have some relevance because
evolution plays an important role in shaping the surfaces of biological creatures, but the reliable indicators of species membership are
deeper properties such as embryonic features and genetic structure.
This is why biologists are confident in saying that humans and
chimps are near relatives, whereas dolphins and salmon are not. And
essentialism applies to the natural world more generally. If you want
to know whether something really is gold, don't just look at it hard;
ask a chemist about its atomic structure.

Or consider medicine. Diagnosis of illness consists of moving
away from surface description to deeper classifications. If you have a
rash, you will be unhappy if a doctor says that it looks "a lot like a
sunburn" and leaves it at that. You want to know what it really is;
this is why we have diagnostic procedures such as blood tests and
biopsies. Or consider some recent developments in oncology. Can-
cers are typically categorized on the basis of the part of the body
they come from—the breast, colon, lung, and so on. But scientists
are developing a better taxonomy based on the genes and proteins
that are responsible for the origin of the tumor. Because this taxonomy is "deeper," it is leads to more accurate prognosis and treatment. Deep is good, and it is essentialism that drives us to search for
the deeper nature of things.

BAD ESSENTIALISM

Essentialism comes in various strengths. I have been talking so far about the version endorsed by John Locke. In previous work, I have described this as "essentialism lite," to contrast it with the much stronger version, articulated in Plato's *Republic* and elaborated by Aristotle, which proposes the existence of ideal, permanent, sharply defined, immutable types. The general consensus among philosophers and scientists is that this strong form of essentialism is invalid, at least for biological categories such as species. As Ernst Mayr, a philosopher of science, grumbled, "It took more than two thousand years for biology, under the influence of Darwin, to escape the paralyzing grip of essentialism."

The most serious consequence of what I will call bad essentialism concerns how we think about race and ethnicity. A mild form of essentialism here makes sense—the surface appearance of people, such as height and skin color, is the result of physiological factors, and to some extent genetic ones. Furthermore, our commonsense characterization of race corresponds roughly to patterns of shared inheritance; gene frequencies do differ slightly across groups that we normally describe as being different races. This is because races are best seen as extended and partly inbred families. As with families, there are fuzzy boundaries, arbitrary cutoffs, and bizarre inclusions and exclusions. But like families, racial groupings tell us something about the likelihood of possessing certain genes. This is why race is relevant for diagnosis of some medical conditions (sickle-cell anemia is more common in blacks; Tay-Sachs disease is more common in Jews). Thus it is reasonable for members of minority groups to lobby for inclusion in medical research.

On the other hand, racial categories do not capture deep discontinuities in the biological world. They do not define distinct subspecies or lineages, and the genetic difference between members of different groups is quite minimal. This is what biologists and anthropologists mean when they say that there is "no such thing" as race.

In addition, racial categorization is greatly influenced by social and cultural factors. Does the son of a Jewish father and Catholic mother count as a Jew? (What if the mother undergoes conversion?) If one parent is from Africa and the other from Mexico, are the children black or Hispanic? If one person is from Haiti and the other from Kenya, do they belong to the same race? These questions have clear answers in many cultures, but the answers are determined by cultural factors, not scientific ones. For example, in the United States the "one drop of blood" rule was used to decide whether a person counted as black.

There is an important sense, then, in which races are artifacts—that is, the concept of race has been created by people, not by nature. But we do not tend to see it this way. Instead, we see race, like species, as corresponding to deeper objective facts about reality. In a national survey, Americans were asked whether they agreed with this statement: "TWO PEOPLE from the SAME RACE will always be more genetically similar to each other than TWO PEOPLE from DIFFERENT RACES." Most adults agreed with this statement. But it is not true. (To see why, consider again the notion that races are like families. Is my child more genetically similar to every other Bloom than to every other non-Bloom, including his mother?) In fact, two randomly chosen members of the same race are genetically far more different from each other than the average member of one race is from the average member of another. The same trend toward bad essentialism shows itself when adults assume that there is an objective fact of the matter as to whether or not someone is *really* Jewish, black, Chinese, Arab, and so on, as well as in the corresponding assumption that each person falls into just a single such category.

Unfortunately, race is actually one of the clearest examples of the natural essentialism of children. An essential notion of race shows up even in three-year-olds. They take a category that is largely determined by social practice, and they treat it as a thing of nature. This in turn sets the foundation for differential treatment of people. As a consequence of stereotyping, for instance, it so happens that in the United States a person's skin color really *is* a strong predictor of all sorts of hidden properties, such as the person's income, educational achievement, and likelihood of being the victim of a violent crime. With regard to human groups, essentialism is a self-fulfilling prophecy. As the anthropologist Lawrence Hirschfeld puts it, "Race is not simply a bad idea; it is a deeply rooted bad idea."

TWENTY THOUSAND KINDS OF ARTIFACTS

I started with categories that are purely natural, such as water, and drifted to those that are permeated by social considerations. Let me take this further to categories that are purely artificial. Consider this excerpt from Tim O'Brien's novel, *The Things They Carried,* set in Vietnam:

> The things they carried were largely determined by necessity. Among the necessities or near-necessities were P-38 can openers, pocket knives, heat tabs, wristwatches, dog tags, mosquito repellent, chewing candy, cigarettes, salt tablets, packets of Kool-Aid, lighters, matches, sewing kits, Military Payment Certificates, C rations, and two or three canteens of water. Together, these items weighed between 15 and 20 pounds, depending on a man's habits or rate of metabolism. Henry Dobbins, who was a big man, carried extra rations; he was especially fond of canned peaches in heavy syrup over pound cake. Dave Jensen, who practiced field hygiene, carried a toothbrush, dental floss, and several hotel-sized bars of soap he'd

stolen on R&R in Sydney, Australia. Ted Lavender, who was scared, carried tranquilizers.

The grunts in this novel are tramping through a jungle, a natural environment if ever there was one. But everything they carry has been created by people. They live in a world of artifacts.

So do you. If you doubt this, go ahead—touch something that is not an artifact. Maybe this is easy; perhaps you are reading this book naked on a desert island. But more likely you are sitting on a chair, lying on a bed, or standing, with a floor beneath your feet. If there is a window, you see roads, lawns, and buildings. If you are eating, the food in front of you—a bagel and coffee, say—has been put together with a process of design no different from the one that produced the bag in which you carried the bagel, or the cup that contains the coffee.

About 1.5 million species have been identified and described so far, an impressive number, but the number of patents in the United States alone is much greater: over 7 million. One psychologist has estimated that we encounter in our lives twenty thousand different kinds of artifacts—far more than the number of different kinds of species we would ever encounter. This diversity of human-made kinds is not entirely a new development; Karl Marx, in 1867, was astonished to hear that five hundred different types of hammers were produced in Birmingham, England, each for a subtly different purpose.

Furthermore, many of the objects in the world that might seem natural are just as artificial as anything that comes out of a factory or can be bought in a store. Wheat and corn, for instance, are new forms of life and need human assistance for their sustenance; corn was carefully bred from a wild grass, and if people were to be whisked off the planet for a few thousand years, corn would cease to exist. Cats began to be bred about ten thousand years ago by the Egyptians, who brought them into their houses and gave them the name *miaw*. Dogs were bred from wolves. (This type of breeding for docility is easier than you might think. In a recent Russian experiment, it took just 15 generations to successfully breed docile foxes that liked being petted, came when called, barked like dogs, and wagged their tails.) We have also bred certain subspecies, such as cats with no hair and pigs with extra pork chops. It is notable that the crude "natural" definition of species—two animals belong to the same species if and only if they can mate and produce viable offspring—does not work for dogs, which can mate with coyotes and timber wolves. What makes a dog a dog has much to do with domesticity, with how we typically interact with it.

You might object that Fido is not an artifact. He is a living thing, flesh and bones. Dogs are born, not made. But we have to be wary of setting up a false dichotomy here. A metal statue is both an artifact that is created by a person, and a physical object that takes up space and is subject to gravity; it is not just one or the other. When the Elephant Man howled, "I am *not* an animal!" he was being imprecise; he should have howled, "I am not *merely* an animal!" Similarly, an object might be both an artifact and a biological entity. Bill Bryson nicely captures the notion that there are two ways of thinking about cows: "To my mind, the only possible pet is a cow. Cows love you. . . . They will listen to your problems and never ask a thing in return. They will be your friends forever. And when you get tired of them, you can kill and eat them."

Finally, there are categories that are artifacts because human goals and interests determine their boundaries. This is the case for dogs. What counts as a dog is partially determined by our own interests, by what we *say* is a dog (quite apart from the fact that humans have guided the biological evolution of dogs). This is true as well for categories such as flowers, grass, herbs, weeds, and trees. These do not correspond to objects that share a common microstructure. They are instead groupings of organisms that share certain humanly relevant properties, such as size and taste. The English word "tree," for instance, refers to a biologically diverse set of plants. From a botanical point of view there is no such thing as a tree. Sometimes an artifact category can exist side by side with a biological one. The classic example of this brings us back to tomatoes. Are they fruits or vegetables? The United States Supreme Court actually ruled on this issue in 1893. (In New York at the time, imported fruits were not taxed, but imported vegetables were, so the status of tomatoes had to be resolved.) The ruling acknowledged that "technically" they are fruit—they are the sex organs of a plant. But "in the common language of the people," tomatoes, along with cucumbers, squashes, beans, and peas, are vegetables, because they are usually served at dinner with the main part of the meal, as opposed to eaten for desert. The verdict was that the tomato is a vegetable. Categories can lead double lives; they can be construed as either natural kinds or as artifacts, kinds bounded by human interest.

ARTIFACT ESSENTIALISM

Returning to more typical examples of artifacts, when we read the list of what O'Brien's soldiers are carrying, we immediately know what the things are. In the real world, we have little problem identifying can openers, knifes, and dental floss—we know what they look like. The simple theory of artifact categories ends here, by proposing that we have some mental representation of what such things look like, and this is what we use when figuring out which category a new object belongs to.

But this theory fails. Consider chairs and clocks. It is easy enough to imagine what typical members of these categories look like, and most of us could even draw crude sketches. But there are beanbag chairs, deck chairs, chairs for dolls, chairs shaped like hands, and chairs suspended from ceilings by chains. There are grandfather clocks, digital clocks, clocks shaped like Coke bottles or handguns, and clocks for the blind that have no visible clock face at all, just buttons and a speaker. In the course of your life, you will be exposed to an extraordinary array of chairs and clocks. Some will be the result of new technology—you might see a hoverchair, a chair that floats above the ground on a cushion of air; perhaps there will be clocks that are embedded in the visual cortex. Other chairs and clocks might be the result of fashion, aesthetics, or just fun. What makes them all chairs and clocks does not depend on their appearance.

An alternative way of assigning objects to categories is based on what these things are used for: chairs are objects that people sit on; clocks are objects that tell time. But this does not work either. If I sit on the table, it is still a table, not a chair, and a fragile chair that cannot hold someone's weight is still a chair. I can tell the time, roughly, by looking at the shadow of a tree, but neither the tree nor the shadow is a clock. And a clock that cannot give the time because it is broken or has no batteries is still a clock. More generally, although artifacts usually have functions, something can be a member of an artifact category even if it doesn't have the typical function. Someone might build a chair just for pleasure, and never sit on it.

We can better explain our intuitive ability to assign objects to the correct category once we realize that essentialism is not limited to the natural world. It applies to artifacts as well. For natural kinds, the essence is seen as some internal property; for artifacts, the essence is seen as the creator's intention. We categorize something as a chair if what it does and what it looks like are best explained in terms of someone intending to create something that falls into the same category as other chairs.

The proposal here is that all categories are believed to have essences. The precise nature of these essences can differ; for categories such as tigers, the essence is understood to be a hidden physical property; for categories such as chairs, it is understood to be the goals and beliefs and desires of the object's creator. This proposal explains certain similarities between how we think about natural things and how we think about artifacts.

1. The superficial parts and properties of animals can be explained to some extent by internal essences such as genetic structure. Similarly, the superficial parts and properties of artifacts can be explained to some extent by intentional essences such as the goals underlying their creation. People have hands because of our genes; clocks have hands because of the function that they are typically intended to fulfill.

2. Appearances are relevant to categorization of both natural kinds and artifacts. We can categorize animals because there is a pretty reliable relationship between appearance and essences. If it looks, walks, and smells like a tiger, an excellent first guess is that it is a tiger. Biological analyses are not necessary. For artifacts, too, appearance and function are reliably linked to the reason the artifact was created. As Daniel Dennett notes, "There can be little doubt what an axe is, or what a telephone is for; we hardly need to consult Alexander Graham Bell's biography for clues about what he had in mind."

3. Intuitions about essence can help us place unusual cases of both natural kinds and artifacts—such as novel and futuristic objects, transformed animals, and bizarre hybrids—in the right category.

4. Finally, in the case of both natural kinds and artifacts, the underlying essence is sometimes hard to find, and so we appeal to experts. For natural kinds, we seek out experts in the fields of genetics, chemistry, and embryology; experts on artifacts are archaeologists, anthropologists, and historians.

The same sort of essentialist biases that children exhibit in the domain of natural kinds show up for artifacts. Several experiments have found that even young children rely on a notion of the creator's intent when they are deciding how to name and categorize artifacts. Other studies show that children are more attuned to the function an artifact was *intended* to fulfill than the function that the artifact actually does fulfill.

In one recent experiment, the psychologist Susan Gelman and I showed children actual objects such as a sharp piece of plastic or a piece of leather that were crafted to look roughly like familiar artifacts such as a knife, or a belt. Then we told the children stories about them. In some of the stories the objects had been created on purpose, and in others they were the results of an accident.

One of the stories about the piece of plastic went like this: "Sam bought a piece of plastic. He got out his saw and carefully sawed the plastic. Then he made it all smooth with sandpaper. Then he was done. This is what it looked like. What is it?"

The other story went like this: "Sam had a piece of plastic. He dropped it and it broke into lots of different pieces. He said, 'Oh, no!' Then he picked up one of the pieces off the floor. This is what it looked like. What is it?"

As predicted, even three-year-olds, who were the youngest who could be tested using this method, were more likely to name the object as a knife if it was described as intentionally created, as in the first story, than if it was described as accidentally created, as in the second. When an artifact is being named, intention matters.

DIVINE ARTIFACTS

Our capacity for mindreading has evolved for making sense of the actions of people, and so we naturally apply it when making sense of the objects people create. This explains why even young children are essentialist toward artifacts. What is perhaps more surprising is that this artifact essentialism—our propensity to think about things in terms of design and purpose—is not limited to actual artifacts. We often extend it as well to the natural world, seeing animals and plants as if they were the products of intentional design.

The notion that the natural world is the handiwork of a divine creator is a common theme across religions. Jews and Christians believe that God willed the world into existence in seven days by calling different things into existence. Language is particularly important in this creation myth. In one account of creation, after God made the animals he brought them to Adam to be named. Adam "gave names to all the cattle, all the birds of heaven, and all the wild beasts." This act of naming marked the fact that man is the master of all of these creatures. Other religions posit more physical processes on the part of the creator or creators, such as vomiting, procreation, masturbation, and the molding of clay.

Why are these sorts of beliefs so common? A useful place to start looking for the answer is to ask people why they believe in God. Most answers fall into the category of arguments based on good design, natural beauty, perfection, and the complexity of the world or universe. This is known as the "argument from design," and it has been advanced over and over again in human history, by theologians, philosophers, and scientists. In 140 B.C. Cicero wrote: "When we see some example of a mechanism such as a globe or a clock. . . do we doubt that it is the creation of a conscious intelligence? So when we see the movement of the heavenly bodies. . . how can we doubt that these too are not only the works of reason but of a reason which is perfect and divine?"

The best-known version of this argument is made by William Paley in *Natural Theology: or, Evidences of the Existence and Attributes of the Deity, Collected from the Appearances of Nature.* This work is an extended argument that the complexity of the natural world begs for an explanation in terms of intentional design. The passage most often quoted from this work is the following:

In crossing a heath, suppose I pitched my foot against a *stone,* and were asked how the stone came to be there; I might possibly answer, that, for anything I knew to the contrary, it had lain there forever: nor would it perhaps be very easy to show the absurdity of this answer. But suppose I had found a *watch* upon the ground, and it should be inquired how the watch happened to be in that place; I should hardly think of the answer which I had before given, that for anything I knew, the watch might have always been there.

The complexity of the watch, composed of many parts that work together to fulfill a complicated function implies that there must have existed, at some time, and at some place or other, an artificer or artificers, who formed it for the purpose which we find it actually to answer; who comprehended its construction, and designed its use.

In great poetic detail, over many hundreds of pages, Paley describes how the complexity of the physical and biological world is actually much richer than that of artifacts. If you think a watch is complicated, just look at the human eye—a device of stunning complexity. Could such a thing really be an accident? No, argues Paley, any rational person would have to make the same inference for the eye that was made for the watch: that it too was the product of an intelligent creator. This is a powerful argument. It swayed the young Charles Darwin, who had to read Paley to prepare for his B.A. examination at Cambridge and was "charmed and convinced of the long line of argumentation."

Prominent contemporary physicists have put forth a related argument, but for them the evidence of a divine creator is not complex design but simple probability. Apparently our existence is very unlikely. Stephen W. Hawking observes that "if the rate of expansion one second after the Big Bang had been less by one part in 10^{10} the universe would have collapsed after a few million years. If it had been greater by one part in 10^{10} the universe would have been essentially empty after a few million years. In neither case would it have lasted long enough for life to develop." And one explanation for this amazingly unlikely event is intentional planning. Freeman Dyson states, "It almost seems as if the Universe must in some sense have known that we were coming," and Paul Davies concludes that "the laws of the universe have engineered their own comprehension."

Not everyone has been impressed with the argument from design. Some philosophers have worried that it explains a mystery with a mystery: If God created the universe, who created God? Also, some have been less awed with the world as it stands; David Hume called it "very faulty and imperfect compared to a superior standard"—more like a "great vegetable" than an intricate machine.

It is fair to say that some of us, unlike Hume, plainly are too easily impressed. When listing the marvels of divine design, Augustine mentions flatulence: "Some can produce at will odorless sounds from their breech, a kind of singing from the other end." In a Canadian poll people were asked to talk about events that inspired a belief in a benevolent God. Some of the events seemed fairly mundane, including, "I went to someone's house and got a good deal on a power tool that I wanted for a long time."

The main problem with the argument from design is that there is now a theory that can explain complex and adaptive design without positing a divine designer: Darwin's theory of natural selection. But it appears to be remarkably hard for many of us to accept this theory. In the United States, about half of all adults endorse creationist views about the origins of species. One study found that even after taking the relevant anthropology courses, over one third of college undergraduates believed that the Garden of Eden was where the first humans appeared "and that the origin itself was an act of creation as performed by God." The evolutionary biologist Richard Dawkins has written that it almost appears as if "the human brain is specifically designed to misunderstand Darwinism, and to find it hard to believe."

Intuitively, the theory of natural selection has two strikes against it. First, evolutionary theory violates hardcore essentialism, as it conflicts with the notion that species have immutable essences (they do not, they evolve). Second, evolutionary theory is not compatible with our propensity for intentional attribution. The central insight of Darwinian theory is that a purely physical process—the gradual accretion of whatever random variants lead to increased survival and reproduction—can mimic, and often surpass, the efforts of the most thoughtful designer. But this process is highly counterintuitive. It is like quantum physics: we can intellectually grasp it, with considerable effort, but it will never feel right to us. When we see complex structure, it looks like the result of intention—beliefs and goals and desires. We are powerfully drawn to Paley's assertion: design requires a designer.

ARTIFICIALISTS

If our belief in a divine creator has its roots in our innate capacity for mindreading, then even young children should see the world as intentionally designed.

This was the view of Jean Piaget, though for quite different reasons. He proposed that children are too cognitively immature to reason in terms of physical processes. They can only reason about the origins of things in terms of intentional agency, and so they at first assume that natural objects are created by people. Later, once the limits of human agency become clear, they shift to believing in a superhuman entity, something similar to an all-powerful parent. Because of children's tendency to conflate natural things and artifacts, Piaget described them as "artificialists."

Research has shown that Piaget was wrong in thinking that children are severely limited in their understanding of the physical world. Even babies have some understanding of physical processes, such as gravity and movement by contact. They can think about bodies as well as about souls. Also, young children can easily distinguish between things that are made by people and those that are not; there is no stage during which children believe that people created the heavens and the earth.

Nevertheless, there is a profound truth here. Some careful recent studies show that this bias to see intentional design in the natural world does exist for children, more so than for scientifically fluent adults.

The psychologist Deborah Kelemen carried out several experiments in which adults and children were shown different pictures and asked whether it made sense to ask what the depicted thing was for. Adults thought it was sensible to ask "What's it for?" about artifacts such as clocks. They also thought it was sensible to talk about the purpose of the parts of animals such as hands and eyes. But they did not think it was sensible to ask the purpose of nonbiological natural kinds like clouds or of whole animals such as tigers. Children, on the other hand, exhibited what Kelemen calls "promiscuous teleology." They would insist that it is acceptable to ask "What's it for?" for *everything* that she showed them. To a four-year-old, everything looks as if it was created for a purpose.

Not surprisingly, then, they are highly receptive to accounts involving divine intervention. The psychologist Margaret Evans tested the children of Christian fundamentalists and the children of non-fundamentalist parents who endorsed evolutionary theory. She asked them to judge the likelihood of different accounts of where things come from—from human intervention, from God, or from evolution. Her central finding was that children were consistently more creationist than their parents; they were drawn to the God explanation even if the adults who raised them were not.

This should not be taken as a sign of immaturity. It is not children who are unusual, after all. Throughout just about all of human history, some version of creationism has been the commonsense view. Given the argument from design, it is intellectually respectable. Most of all, artificialism is a natural by-product of a mind evolved to think in terms of goals and intentions.

Also, artificialism is emotionally reassuring. It is flattering to believe that the natural world exists for our use, that we have, as Genesis assures us, dominion over "the fish of the sea, the birds of the air, and all the living things that move on the Earth." There is something appealing as well in the idea that we ourselves are the handiwork of a divine creator. Artifacts have purposes, they exist for reasons, and they can be put to proper and improper use. If we are artifacts, then all of this holds true for us. Indeed, religious texts are often explicit as to what these purposes are. In Ecclesiastes we are instructed: "Fear God, and keep his commandments, for this is the whole duty of man."

Artificialism, then, not only is intellectually appealing, meshing well with our evolved stances toward the world, but also exerts considerable emotional pull. One can sympathize with the wife of the bishop of Birmingham, who when she first heard of Darwin's theory, is reputed to have said to her husband, "My dear, let us hope it is not true, but, if it is true, let us hope it will not become generally known."

3

ANXIOUS OBJECTS

Other group members stored their bodily fluids in baby-food jars or wrote cryptic messages on packaged skirt steaks. Their artworks were known as "pieces," a phrase I enthusiastically embraced. "Nice piece," I'd say. In my eagerness to please, I accidentally complimented chipped baseboards and sacks of laundry waiting to be taken to the cleaners. Anything might be a piece if you looked at it hard enough. High on crystal, the gang and I would tool down the beltway, admiring the traffic cones and bright yellow speed bumps. The art world was our conceptual oyster, and we ate it raw.

—David Sedaris, *Twelve Moments in the Life of the Artist*

WHEN THE ART critic James Elkins put an ad in newspapers and journals asking for stories from people who have responded to a painting with tears, he received about four hundred calls, emails, and letters. Some people said that they cried because the paintings depicted awful things, such as loss and loneliness and humiliation. Sometimes the tears were for personal reasons: An English professor told of a painting done by his wife, showing a bed empty and unmade, that was painted right before she had an affair. The professor was looking at it much later, and he suddenly realized that this was their bed, and he thought about what the painting meant, and began to cry.

Artwork can inspire other strong feelings. The art historian E. H. Gombrich told Elkins that he is unable to look at Rembrandt's *Blinding of Sampson*—it is too violent for him to bear. And an Ed Kienholz sculpture had to be removed from display at the Louisiana Museum of Modern Art because it was so revolting that people vomited when they saw it.

These reactions make sense. If watching someone in agony is disturbing, then it naturally follows that it would be disturbing to view a painting that realistically depicts such a scene. And if looking at attractive people, delicious food, nice environments, and happy children is enjoyable, then paintings that resemble these things should give rise to similar feelings of pleasure. In general, once we know what sorts of real-world things inspire certain emotions, it follows that realistic paintings of such things would inspire the very same emotions, though perhaps to a lesser extent.

But it is not that simple. Elkins suggests that the paintings that have prompted the most crying are those by Mark Rothko, in particular, fourteen of them that hang in a chapel in Houston, Texas. The paintings are purplish-black rectangles, not totally black, but uneven, with undulating colors and textures. It is not clear what they represent, if anything. Why would these lead to any emotional response at all? Why would anyone *care* about such things?

Some of our strongest responses to art are elicited by the troubling and controversial modern creations that the art critic Harold Rosenberg has called "anxious objects," artifacts such as these:

- Marcel Duchamp's "ready-mades," objects that were once mere snow shovels and urinals, now transformed into famous artworks.
- Andy Warhol's famous *Brillo Box*, which, although constructed out of plywood, looks much like a box that one could buy in a grocery store.

- Tracey Emin's *My Bed,* which was the actual bed upon which Emin contemplated suicide.
- Maurizio Cattelan's *Novecento* (*Twentieth Century*), which was a dead horse suspended from the ceiling.
- Mark Wallinger's *A Real Work of Art,* which was a living racehorse that the artist was part owner of.
- Francis Alys's *The Ambassador,* which was a live peacock. The work's title refers to the fact that the artist declined to go to the 2001 Venice Biennale, and sent the peacock instead. According to Alys's representatives, "The bird will strut at all the exhibitions and parties, as if he is the artist himself. It is anecdotal, insinuating the vanity of the art world and tying in old animal fables."
- Assorted minimalist works, such as perfectly white canvases, or sculptures that consist of pieces of aluminum, cardboard, or broken glass.

Admittedly, we do not normally weep at such objects; they typically affect our heads more than our hearts. But they do matter to us. They are displayed in museums and galleries; they elicit pleasure and interest and controversy. And some of them are pricey. As I write this, a newspaper reports that an untitled abstract sculpture by Donald Judd sold at Christie's for over $4.6 million, and an Ed Ruscha painting called *Talk About Space,* a blue canvas with the word SPACE written on top in large yellow letters, sold for $3.5 million. These huge sums provide objective evidence that for at least some people these things have *value,* more so than houses, cars, and other utilitarian objects. Why?

In the play *Art,* a dermatologist named Serge buys an expensive piece of modern art, an unframed white canvas with some hard-to-see diagonal scars. His friend Marc is astonished at this choice, and expresses himself with some impatience:

MARC: You paid two hundred thousand francs for this shit?

Later Serge complains to another friend.

SERGE: I don't blame him for not responding to this painting, he hasn't the training, there's a whole apprenticeship you have to go through, which he hasn't, either because he's never wanted to or because he has no particular instinct for it, none of that matters, no, what I blame him for is his tone of voice, his complacency, his tactlessness.

It is fair to say that most art critics, art historians, and artists themselves would take Serge's side of the debate, while many psychologists would be more sympathetic to Marc. Some of these psychologists have argued that, whether they know it or not, those who value such anxious objects do so not for aesthetic reasons but for sociological ones. Steven Pinker makes this point in particularly sharp terms:

> The very uselessness of art that makes it so incomprehensible to evolutionary biology makes it all too comprehensible to economics and social psychology. What better proof that you have money to spare than your being able to spend it on doodads and stunts that don't fill the belly or keep the rain out but that require precious materials, years of practice, a command of obscure texts, or intimacy with the elite? Thorstein Veblen's and Quentin Bell's analyses of taste and fashion, in which an elite's conspicuous displays of consumption, leisure, and outrage are emulated by the rabble, sending the elite off in search of new inimitable displays, nicely explain the otherwise inexplicable oddities of the arts. . . . The value of art is largely unrelated to aesthetics: a priceless masterpiece becomes worthless if it is found to be a forgery; soup cans and comic strips become high art when the art world says they are, and then command conspicuously wasteful

prices. Modern and postmodern works are intended not to give pleasure but to confirm or confound the theories of a guild of critics and analysts, to *épater la bourgeoisie,* or to baffle the rubes in Peoria.

Without denying the force of these social considerations, I want to offer a quite different, though complementary, theory of our understanding and appreciation of these anxious objects. In essence, my goal here is to domesticate modern art, to narrow the gap between certain universal human propensities—particularly those that have to do with how we think about people and the things that people create—and these curious and controversial entities. To do this, I need to start with babies.

BABY PICTURES

The earliest-emerging ability that bears a relationship to art is the ability to appreciate visual representations. Even babies can do this. If you let five-month-olds play with a doll and then take it away and show them pictures of dolls, they will look longer at a picture of a new doll than at one of the doll that they just played with, an indication that they appreciate that an object and a realistic depiction of it are very closely related. When children start to talk, they use words to name not only actual objects, but also objects portrayed in pictures. There is also some dramatic evidence that—contrary to some anthropological anecdotes—naming pictured objects does not require any prior experience with pictures. In 1962, the psychologists Julian Hochberg and Virginia Brooks reported a study where they took a child (presumably their own, though they did not say) and raised him without any access to pictures, television, or other visual representations. Then, when he was 19 months old, they showed him a series of photographs and line drawings of familiar objects and asked him to name them. He did so easily.

Who would have thought otherwise? After all, both Euclid and Leonardo da Vinci pointed out that a realistic painting works because it can impress upon the eye much the same visual array as the real world. A realistic picture of a dog looks to the eye much like a real dog. In fact, with *trompe l'oeil* ("fool the eye") artwork one actually cannot tell the difference between representation and reality. There is a story by O. Henry about a sickly woman who says that she will die when the last leaf falls. She stares out the window of her apartment, and after all the other leaves fall, one remains, even as the season changes. The leaf turns out to have been painted on the brick wall opposite by an elderly painter who wants to keep her alive. The ability to recognize realistic pictures is nothing more than a by-product of how vision works. Any creature that gets information through the senses—any creature that is not a deity—runs the risk of being confused by a clever enough representation.

(The opposite error—taking the real thing for a representation—is rare, but it does happen. At a masquerade ball in Monte Carlo there was a competition to decide which of the guests masquerading as Charlie Chaplin looked most like Chaplin. It so happened that Chaplin himself was there. He got third prize.)

It is possible, then, that babies might be able to recognize pictures without any understanding of their role as representations. And, in fact, children younger than about one and a half years of age do seem confused by pictures. Attentive adults have noticed certain weird behaviors such as a child trying to step into a picture of a shoe or scratching at a picture book as if trying to grasp the object depicted there. When experimenters plunk babies down in front of picture books and film their behavior, it turns out that they really do tend to treat depicted objects as if they were real, and try to lift them from the page. This is not limited to children living within representation-rich Western culture; those from impoverished and illiterate families in the Ivory Coast, where pictures are rare, do the same thing.

Babies can tell objects and pictures apart. When given the choice, they prefer to look at a doll than a picture of a doll; and they reach for real objects more often than they reach for pictures of objects. Also, when they try to pick up a depicted object and fail, they are not *that* upset; they seem somewhat resigned to their failure. It seems likely that they are confused about what pictures are; they are seen as bizarre things, as inferior objects—like real things in shape and color, but strangely flat. As the psychologist Judy DeLoache and her colleagues put it, "They treat a depiction as though it were an object, not because they firmly believe it is, but because they are unsure that it is not."

Adults are smarter than this; we know that pictures are representations and can be used as a medium to understand and talk about the things they represent. When someone shows you a picture of her child, she doesn't expect you to admire the *picture*; when she says "This is Emma," she is not naming regions of pixels or two-dimensional patterns of color. Much of what we know about the external world is not learned through seeing the things themselves, but by seeing pictures of them.

Indeed, most of us learn about specific artworks not by looking at the works but by looking at *pictures* of the works. (Almost everyone knows what the *Mona Lisa* looks like but only a small minority has actually seen it.) You might think, following Plato, that the original is always better than the representation, but this might not be true. One of Elkins's criers wept because of disappointment. Entranced by a film about Michelangelo's work, she flew to Florence and felt horribly let down by what she saw: "The statues were not as great as the *photographs* of them!"

WOULD YOU EAT
A PICTURE OF AN APPLE?

By the time children are about a year and a half, they no longer reach for pictures. Do they then appreciate their representational nature? To explore this, the psychologists Susan Carey and Melissa Allen Preissler did a simple but elegant study. They used pictures to teach children new words. For instance, they would take 18-month-olds who had never seen a whisk before, show them a line drawing of a whisk, and repeatedly use the word "whisk" to describe the drawing. Then they would give the children a choice between the very same picture they were trained on and a real whisk and ask them to find "the whisk." Children almost always go for the actual object. This is quite neat. It shows that they know that when a name is used for a picture, it does not refer to the picture itself; it refers to what the picture represents. Before children reach their second birthday, then, they know what pictures are.

I should admit that not all psychologists would agree with this. Some research purports to show that even older children are deeply confused about representations. Three-year-olds will sometimes say yes when asked, "Can you eat this picture of an apple?" They will sometimes agree that if you get close to a picture of a rose, you can smell it. Some of them will even agree that if you cut a picture of a rattle in half, something would happen to the real rattle! Other studies find that when asked to "point to things you can really eat," young children pointed not only to real foods, but also to pictures of food—even if they had previously agreed that the pictures are "just pictures."

Some researchers take this as showing a failure to distinguish reality from representation. I am skeptical. I think it just shows that children can be misled by weird questions. Adults are savvy enough about what goes on in a psychology experiment to focus on the literal form of what they are asked and to ignore normal rules of conversation. Imagine how strange it would be to be shown a picture of some food and be asked, "Can you eat it?" and assume that the person was asking about the *picture*. We do sometimes ask about pictures for their own sake, but this is typically if they are themselves of some artistic merit, as when a German officer once handed Picasso a postcard of his painting *Guernica*—inspired by the German bomb-ing of the Basque village of that name—and asked, "Did you do that?" Picasso replied, "No, you did."

If these older children really didn't understand pictures, you would expect them to act oddly toward them in everyday life, but they don't. They might say that you can eat a picture of an apple, but if you ask them to go ahead and do so, they decline. Finally, children surely don't *really* think that what happens to a picture happens to the object. As the psychologist Norman Freeman pointed out, if you tell a three-year-old you are going to tear up a picture of her, she will not be struck with mortal terror.

This is not to say that young children are fully competent with representations. Some of their limitations are obvious: they cannot read maps, flowcharts, diagrams, and, most important, words. All this has to be learned.

Also, DeLoache and her colleagues have discovered that children have problems coping with the "dual nature" of representations—the fact that they are both concrete entities and abstract symbolic ones. For instance, two-and-a-half-year-olds can use a picture of a room to re-cover the location of a hidden toy. Once they see where the toy is in the picture, they know where to find it in the room itself. But they do much worse when shown the location of the toy in a three-dimensional model. This is surprising, because you might think that a model, being more realistic, would be easier to make sense of than a picture, and easier to use as a representation. But DeLoache argues that the model is so interesting (it is a tangible three-dimensional object) that children focus on it as a thing in itself, and this distracts them from its representational properties. When the model is made less in-teresting, children become better able to use it to find the hidden toy.

These findings have important practical implications. In cases of suspected sexual abuse, investigators often use anatomically correct dolls to try to elicit accurate reporting of what happened to the children. But there is some evidence that, at least with two- and three-year-olds, this is useless and misleading because dolls are sufficiently interesting in their own right that children fail to understand that they are supposed to serve as representations—in this case, of human bodies.

Adults shouldn't be too smug. We also do better when not distracted by extraneous properties of representations. And we can sometime confuse a change in representation with a change in reality, getting muddled about what happens when one shifts to and from daylight savings time or moves from one time zone to another. A dramatic example of this is when England adopted the Georgian calendar on September 3, 1752, which caused that date suddenly to become September 14. Farmers rioted because they worried that the lost 11 days would ruin the growing season!

MAKING AND NAMING PICTURES

Every culture has some form of art, if only scratches on trees, markings on cave walls, or drawings in the sand. And all normal humans have some capacity to create art. Children love to draw, scribble, and mold with clay. There are plainly cultural and individual differences, but this should not obscure the universal tendency to make and appreciate art.

What can we learn from the earliest creations of children who have been raised in Western cultures? The most obvious fact is that these creations are not, to put it mildly, realistic. The psychologist Howard Gardner begins his book *Artful Scribbles* by giving us a tour of children's drawings and comparing each one to the work of a renowned adult artist. Here is Danny, whose minimalist creations are reminiscent of those of Theo van Doesburg; Kathy's painting looks much like the work of Jackson Pollock; this painting by Thomas could have well been done by Miró, Picasso, or Klee. These are all *abstract* artists; nobody says of children that they draw like Rembrandt, da Vinci, or Vermeer.

It might seem that even if these early creations are sensibly thought of as art, they are not representational art; they are not about anything in the world. But there is one wrinkle here: *Children name their creations.* They describe their scribbles, scrawls, and blotches using ordinary terms such as "Mommy," "truck," and so on. I first became interested in the psychology of art when my son Max, then a two-year-old, pointed to some smears of paint and proudly said that it was "an airplane."

What should we conclude from this behavior? Does Max believe that his paint blob represents an airplane? Do other children believe that their scribbles represent trucks, horses, their mothers? Gardner considers this issue, and raises several possibilities:

> Does the child really discern a resemblance that happens to be missed by everyone else? Does he seek to "wish" the form into being by so anointing it; might he even be performing some kind of magical or totemistic act? Does the child see labeling as a game in which the culture participates, or is it done simply to please adults who may well have been bombarding him with the inevitable "What is it? What are you drawing? Tell me what it is."

Although Gardner goes on to entertain the notion that there is *some* representational ability displayed here—perhaps the marks are "a primitive kind of notation standing for the object"—he is ultimately unsympathetic to this view and goes on to dub children's naming "romancing" because the child's names "promise representations which are not, however, delivered." If there is representational intent here, it is not successful.

But consider a different possibility, which is that children are representational artists from the moment they put crayon to paper. If

so, then the child's perspective corresponds to that of the narrator of
the classic children's book *The Little Prince,* which begins with his
thinking about jungle adventures, and then creating a simple col-
ored drawing, a brown shape that looks like a hat. He then shows it
to adults and asks if they are frightened. They reply, "Why be scared
of a hat?" The child writes, "My drawing was not a picture of a hat.
It was a picture of a boa constrictor digesting an elephant." Later,
discouraged, the narrator notes, "Grown-ups never understand anything by themselves, and it is exhausting for children to have to provide explanations over and over again."

What makes the brown shape a snake swallowing an elephant,
presumably, is that the child intends it to be so. Perhaps, then, for a
child, if something is *intended* to represent a thing, then it *does* represent that thing and can be given that name.

If this is true, it would follow that, at a minimum, children
should be able to name pictures that do not resemble what they
depict. This is what I explored in collaboration with the psychologist Lori Markson. In one study, three- and four-year-olds were
told that they were going to be shown some pictures drawn by a
child their own age who had a broken arm. To explain why the
pictures were so unrealistic, they were informed that the child
tried *really* hard to draw good pictures, but because of the broken
arm, the pictures did not always come out looking like what the
child wanted.

In the "size task," the children were shown a drawing that depicted two squiggles of unequal size and were told, "She drew a picture of a spider and a tree." In the "oddity task," they were shown a
drawing of four ovals, one with a different orientation than the rest,
and told, "She drew three pigs and one chicken." During testing,
the experimenter pointed to each figure in the picture and asked the
children to describe it. This is easy enough for an adult. For the size
task, we take the relative sizes of the markings to correspond to the

relative sizes of the objects in the world, and name the smaller object as the spider and the larger one as the tree. For the oddity task, we assume that the markings that look the same correspond to objects of the same kind, and the one that looks different corresponds to the object of a different kind, and so we correctly label the three pigs and the one chicken.

We found that even three-year-olds did better than chance on both tasks. They can name pictures on the basis of cues other than resemblance. This fits with the results of another study that used two yellow Ping-Pong balls of identical size, but one much heavier than the other. Children were told, "I have a daddy and a baby." On some trials they were asked to point to "the daddy"; on others they were asked to point to "the baby." By the age of about two and a half, children succeeded at picking the heavy one as the daddy.

The next step was to directly explore whether children of this age could actually use the intent of a person when making sense of drawings. To test this, we did a study where two similar objects, such as a fork and a spoon, were placed in front of the child, one to the left and one to the right. The experimenter looked intently at one of the objects and appeared to draw a picture of it. Unbeknownst to the child, the picture had actually been predrawn to look equally like both of the objects.

The picture was then placed between the two objects and the child was asked what it was a picture of. Almost always, the answer depended on what the child thought the experimenter was intending to draw. If she had been looking at the spoon while "drawing" it, they called it "a spoon"; if she was looking at the fork, they called it "a fork." The very same picture got a different name according to how the child thought it had been created.

We then did a similar version with pictures that children themselves drew. Children were requested to draw four pictures on separate sheets of paper, each with a different-colored crayon. These were

(1) a balloon, (2) a lollipop, (3) the child him- or herself, (4) the experimenter. After a pause of several minutes during which the child and the experimenter engaged in another activity, the experimenter "rediscovered" the drawings and asked the child to describe them.

The logic behind this study is that preschool children are notoriously unskilled artists. By having them draw different pictures of entities similar in appearance, we reasoned that their subsequent naming of these pictures could not be based on appearance, but would have to be determined, at least in part, by their memory of their own representational intent. It is important to note that, as expected, the drawings often did not look anything like balloons, lollipops, or people, and even when they did—mostly for the four-year-olds—one could not tell from its appearance whether a given drawing represented a lollipop or a balloon or the experimenter or the child. A typical example from a four-year-old is shown in figure 3.1.

As predicted, when later asked to name the drawings, both the three-year-olds and four-year-olds did so on the basis of what they had intended them to represent. If they created their drawing with the intent that it should represent a balloon, they would call it a balloon; if they wanted it to be a lollipop, they would call it a lollipop. This is not a subtle laboratory phenomenon: a good way to make a child cry is to take a picture that is described as "Mommy" and insist that it is a picture of someone else—the child's brother, say. Children resent this; they know it is a picture of Mommy because that is the person they intend it to depict.

If understanding pictures requires understanding people's goals and desires, it follows that autistic children should have problems understanding pictures.

They do. Melissa Allen Preissler gave autistic children the "whisk study" described earlier, where the experimenter named a picture of a novel object and then tested whether children would later extend

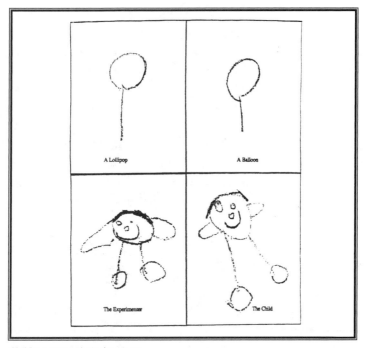

Children name their drawings.

FROM BLOOM AND MARKSON, "CHILDREN'S NAMING OF REPRESENTATIONS," *PSYCHOLOGICAL SCIENCE*, APRIL 1997, 4-6, BY PERMISSION OF BLACKWELL PUBLISHING.

the name to the same picture or the real object that the picture depicts. She found that unlike the normally developing children, autistic children would choose the picture.

What about much older and more adept autistic individuals? In some research that I did in collaboration with the psychologists Frances Abell, Francesca Happé, and Uta Frith, we explored whether they could use the intention of the artist when naming pictures. We tested older autistic children, of an average age of about 10 years old, and a verbal IQ of about 7 years old. These were reasonably well functioning individuals; you could converse with them, and they had no problem naming objects in realistic pictures which actually resembled what they depicted. Our first effort was to duplicate the study that Lori Markson and I had done with pictures of lollipops, balloons, and the experimenter. We asked our autistic subjects to draw these things and later asked them to name them, predicting that they would not be able to tap their memory of their original intent to do so.

This experiment was a disaster. The problem was that the logic of the study rested on the children creating pictures that could not be named on the basis of appearance—and our subjects were just too adroit at drawing. Their lollipops looked like lollipops; their pictures of me (when I was the experimenter) looked like me. In retrospect, this should not have been that surprising, given that autistic children tend to be good artists. But it meant that the study could not be done, since our subjects could name their drawings without any appeal to intention, just by looking at them.

So we did something else. The child sat across from the experimenter, with either four toy cars or four toy planes spread in a line between them. The objects differed in color but were otherwise identical. The experimenter looked intently at one of the objects, drew it using a pencil, and then asked the child, "What is this a picture of?" In another task, using a different display of identical objects, the subjects were given a piece of paper and a pencil and asked to draw any one of the objects. Then the experimenter asked what their picture was of. Correct responses in both tasks entailed identifying the precise object that was attended to (by either the experimenter or by the subject) as the picture was being drawn. If a subject gave a vague answer, such as "A car" or "A plane," he or she was asked "Which car?" or "Which plane?" Note that because the only differentiating feature was color, the target of the drawing could not be identified by resemblance. The child would have to look at the drawing and remember the intention behind it.

For the sake of comparison, we also tested a group of normally developing children. These were younger than the autistic children, they had, on average, a lower verbal IQ, and they were nowhere near as good as drawing pictures. But they had no impairment in social reasoning.

We found that the children with autism performed significantly less well than the normally developing children, both when naming the picture drawn by the experimenter and when naming the picture that they themselves had drawn. These autistic children did not seem to have the same instinctive understanding about the relationship between what a picture was or how it should be named and the intent of the artist—even when they themselves were the artists.

BUT IS IT ART?

The discussion so far has been about the emerging understanding of representations. But not all art is representational, and not all representations are artwork. The question then arises: What sorts of things do children—and adults—think of as art?

A skeptic might worry there is no limit to the things that can be art and there is no property that they all share. What does a painting by Rembrandt or a sculpture by Henry Moore have in common with Duchamp's urinal or Wallinger's horse? What properties do these share with John Cage's *4'33"*, which is performed by a pianist who just sits, without moving, at a piano for 4 minutes, 33 seconds? Or consider "performance art" such as the works of Chris Burden, which involve his being placed in a canvas bag in the middle of a busy California street (*Deadman*), crawling through broken glass (*Through the Night Softly*), and being placed on the shelf of an art gallery for several days without food and water (*White Light/White Heat*). These sorts of unusual cases are not necessarily modern: the

Roman emperor Heliogabalus was said to have slaughtered slaves on the lawn because their blood mingled beautifully with the green grass. This is clearly immoral. But is it art?

Also, art is a self-conscious endeavor, and so an attempt to define art is likely to inspire a clever artist to react with a counterexample. In fact, many modern works of art have the goal of shocking the world by saying: *This too is art.* Some philosophers conclude that, in the end, art is nothing more than whatever the right people (artists, critics, gallery owners, and so on) say it is.

But this skeptical position cannot be entirely right. People have gut feelings about the matter. We instinctively judge some things as definitely art, others as definitively not art, and still others as fuzzy or indeterminate cases. We can make these judgments on the basis of hearing how the objects were created or by observing their creation—we do not have to wait for the authorities to come to a verdict. We have, in our heads, then, some notion of what art is.

Consider also some of the things that children create. They will often collect interesting natural objects or artifacts and display them in special ways, and I'm not sure that it is too much of a stretch to see this as akin to Duchamp's "ready-mades." My son Zachary, who is four, creates what he calls "experiments." He takes objects from around the house—chairs, socks, cereal—and piles them up in complicated ways, and then proudly brings together his family and visitors to observe and admire them. He does not describe such works as "art," and would be unfamiliar with the term used in such a general sense—but it seems that he invests his creations with a special status, as you and I would if we created works of art.

I propose that what makes art art has to do with particular sorts of intention. Some philosophers suggest that an artwork is something intended to have an audience. This is obvious enough for canonical works, but it also helps with some of the more modern cases discussed earlier. Real Brillo boxes were merely meant as boxes for Brillo, while Warhol's creations were intended to be exhibited. Someone sitting in front of a piano might just be resting or waiting, but Cage's work was meant to be *performed*. And there is a world of difference between crawling through broken glass out of necessity or madness, and doing so in front of an audience. When a child creates an artwork, as with Zachary's "experiments," he or she typically expects to show it to others.

As the philosophers are well aware, this idea that what makes something art is its creator's intention that it have an audience cannot be exactly right, since some artists, such as Franz Kafka and Emily Dickinson, created their work with the express intention that it *not* have an audience. So the definition has to be modified somewhat; perhaps an artwork is something that is intended to be the sort of thing that *normally* has an audience. And this is presumably why Kafka and Dickinson made a point of telling people to destroy their work, because they recognized that otherwise it would be shown to others. A more difficult problem with this theory is that not everything intended to have an audience counts as art (this book, for instance). And so this theory has to be further modified, perhaps by sharpening the notion of what an audience is or of precisely how the work is presented.

One particularly promising theory along these lines has been developed by the philosopher Jerrold Levinson, who suggests that art is something created with the intent that it be seen in a certain way—"as art objects in the present or past are correctly regarded." In other words, we judge something to be an artwork if we believe that it was intended to be seen in the same way that we see other, already existing, artwork.

This captures our intuitions nicely. It explains why we see paintings, sculpture, and music as art. It captures the difference between *In Advance of a Broken Arm* and a snow shovel, a drunken prank and a stylish work of performance art, an accidental spill and an abstract painting, and so on. It allows us to capture the connectedness of art through history (the art of any period is rooted in the art prior to it, so if something was art in the past it should still be art now), while at the same time accounting for the existence of an ever-broadening notion of art (if the art of a given period is based and built upon prior art, then it follows that the scope of art can increase).

Finally, this notion of art is immune to innovations by artists. It is easy enough to see how an artist might rebel against the notion that art has to do with beauty, or representation, or the arousing of certain emotions—and there is plenty of art that defies these theories because they aren't beautiful, they are not representational, they do not arouse those emotions. But Levinson's definition is bulletproof—once an artist makes something with the intent that it be seen as an artwork, then it is an artwork.

Is this how children understand art? We know from the studies reviewed earlier that children use intention when deciding what to call certain drawings. In a recent series of experiments, the psychologists Susan Gelman and Karen Ebeling have explored the more general question of whether children are sensitive to intention when deciding whether or not something is an artwork.

Two- and three-year-olds were shown a series of simple drawings. Half of the children were told that these depicted intentional creations. For instance, they were shown a drawing in the shape of a man and told: "When John was painting in art class, he used some paint to make something for his teacher. This is what it looked like." The rest of the children were told that it was an accidental creation: "When John's dad was painting the house, John accidentally spilled some paint on the floor. This is what it looked like." They were then asked, "What is this?" Children who had been told that the shape was created on purpose were more likely to say "A man"— that is, to name the depicted object. Children who had been told that it was accidentally created often answered with a description of the material that was used: "Paint." In other words, the mode of creation makes a difference: children appear to treat the intentionally created object, but not the accidentally created one, as an artwork.

Gelman and Ebeling worried that in this study the cues to the creator's intent are all supplied verbally; children are explicitly told how the objects are created. It is neither natural nor subtle. So they did another study where they showed two-year-olds videotapes of artwork being created. For instance, they would see someone act as if she inadvertently squirted yellow paint on a paper (roughly in the shape of the sun); this would be reinforced by the character's shouting "Oh no!" In another videotape, the same woman would carefully create the artwork, faintly smiling, intently working on it, and saying "Good" at the end. Again, as predicted, two-year-olds got the difference, being more likely to name the painting (as "sun," for instance) when it was shown to be created on purpose. In art, intention counts.

ART AND OTHER ARTIFACTS

This theory of how we name and categorize art is a natural extension of the theory presented in the last chapter about more mundane things like clocks and chairs. In both cases, our understanding is rooted in our assumptions about the intent of the creator.

Consider also the creation of art. The traditional way to make an artwork is for the artist to take "raw materials," a lump of clay, perhaps, or oils and a canvas, and impose structure on them, radically modifying them to create a sculpture or painting. This is also the usual way to create a nonartistic artifact, as when we build a chair from pieces of wood. For some artwork, considerable structure is present from the start, as when an artist transforms a preexisting object into art, as in the work of Warhol and Duchamp. But this sort of transformation exists outside the domain of art as well: houses can become churches, crates become bookshelves, computer monitors turn into fish tanks, and swords are beaten into ploughshares.

Some conceptual art is created without any physical manipulation at all, through an act of the artist's imagination. But again, this is true as well for some nonartistic objects. If a chess set is missing a piece, the players can agree to take a penny and make it into a pawn. Indeed, just as with art, the right sort of intention is necessary—a one-year-old cannot turn a penny into a pawn, because she doesn't know about chess. Nevertheless, such transfiguration is not entirely adult business. For instance, children use the word "toy" in this fashion—to refer to things that *they* think of as toys, even if they were not originally intended to be toys.

But there is one way in which art really is different from other objects. All other artifacts are designed for a purpose, but there is nothing less useful than a painting or a sculpture, and the very idea of using one for a functional purpose betrays a misunderstanding. Someone who looks at *In Advance of a Broken Arm*—indistinguishable from a snow shovel—and thinks, "Hmmm, that would help me clear off the driveway this winter," is surely confused. In cold pragmatic terms—to the eyes of a hard-boiled evolutionary psychologist or cultural anthropologist, say—the existence of art is a puzzle. Why do we value such objects?

Part of the answer has to do with the sociological factors I raised at the start of the chapter. Someone might enjoy having an expensive blank white canvas in their living room for much the same reason that Aristotle Onassis is said to have had his barstools upholstered with the scrota of killer whales. It is pleasurable to engage in outrageous, unnecessary, and expensive acts because they serve as displays of status and power, and we are, for reasons having to do with both evolution and culture, constituted so as to enjoy producing such displays.

With regard to certain modern works there is the additional ingredient of displaying intelligence and sophistication. Any moron can gawk at a Rembrandt, but appreciating "anxious objects" requires special expertise. (Recall what Serge said in the play *Art*: "There's a whole apprenticeship you have to go through.") Indeed, some works, such as Sherrie Levine's *Fountain/After Marcel Duchamp* or Mike Bidlo's *Not Andy Warhol (Brillo Box)*, exist as commentary on other modern artworks, and so even their *titles* are understandable only to the elite. Finally, the enjoyment of certain provocative pieces, such as Robert Mapplethorpe's *Self-portrait*, provides a sure sign of one's sophisticated and cosmopolitan nature in sexual and religious matters, just as possession and admiration of more traditional family portraits or religious artworks serve as an advertisement of piety, social standing, and status in the community.

But status is not the only reason we value artworks. On the other extreme, some of the pleasure from art comes from the most basic systems of perception and emotion. Realistic pictures can serve as a substitute, a surrogate, for the real thing. There are certain things we enjoy looking at, and if we cannot have the things themselves (or, for whatever reason, do not want to have them), we will settle for representations. A good painting of a landscape helps to make up for the lack of a view, pictures of flowers can serve as substitutes for real ones. The same goes for pictures of tasty food and naked people.

Also, there are certain formal properties that some art has, aspects of balance and form and color that simply look good to the eye, and it is an ongoing project in the visual sciences to try to explain why. Perhaps surprisingly, this is part of the appeal of some more contemporary artwork. Andres Serrano's famous photograph of a crucifix floating in a golden haze is described by Anthony Julius as having a "blurred, rather conventional beauty" while Louis Menand states that it is "technically and formally, a rather beautiful and evocative piece"—though once you know the title, *Piss Christ*, it

changes the way you see it. Similarly, Mapplethorpe rather inno-
cently remarks that his approach to photography focuses on lighting
and composition, and it is all the same to him whether he is photo-
graphing a flower or a penis.

Then there is the intellectual appeal. Art can give rise to the same
pleasure as an elegant mathematical proof, a clever argument, or a
brilliant insight. Much of modern art comments on the nature of
representation, gender roles, Western and non-Western cultures,
and, of course, art itself. Art blends into philosophy, then, and good
art might give pleasure for the same reason that good philosophy
does. Some take this further and argue that any art that can be immediately understood could not have been that good in the first
place. An article in *ARTnews* ("Baffled, Bewildered—and Smitten:
How to Learn to Stop Worrying and Love the Art You Don't Understand") quotes a curator in the Museum of Modern Art in New
York as saying, "The nature of really serious art is that you don't
know what you're looking at."

But there is an important aspect of the psychology of art that is
missing from this list of reasons for valuing it.

WHAT IS WRONG WITH A FORGERY?

When it was thought to be a painting by Jan Vermeer, *The Supper at
Emmaus* was extremely well regarded, but when it was discovered to
have been painted by the considerably less esteemed twentieth-
century forger Han van Meegeren, its value dropped precipitously.
In fact, according to Dutch law, once the court ruled it to be a forgery it could have been promptly destroyed.

Forgery is just the most dramatic example of the importance of
origin. Arthur Koestler described a friend who owned a drawing that
she first took to be a reproduction. When she later discovered that
it was an original by Picasso, she displayed it more prominently,

claimed that she *saw* it differently, and enjoyed it more. For her, its value went up. To me this makes sense. I love the work of Marc Chagall and would pay plenty for an original painting of his. But I would be a lot less inclined to pay a fortune for a copy—even if I could never tell the difference. I would not enjoy it as much.

Such preferences cannot be explained solely in terms of market forces. It is true that Koestler's friend might reasonably be pleased because now her Picasso is worth more. It is also true that when an artist dies, his or her work rises in value, and that the more copies of a print that are in circulation, the less each one is worth. But financial value is rarely the sole factor in our preference for originals. Presumably most of us would prefer an original even if we have no wish ever to sell it. And anyway, an appeal to economics just pushes the question back: Why would the origin matter to other people—such as potential buyers? Our preferences explain the higher market value of originals, not the other way around.

Cynics have a field day here. When Pinker makes his case for how *non*-aesthetic our appreciation of art is, his first example is that "a priceless masterpiece becomes worthless if it is found to be a forgery." And Koestler claims that the obsession with origin is based on a serious confusion bordering on "fetish worship."

On some accounts, van Meegeren had a similar view. His forgeries were a trap for the critics. The philosopher Alfred Lessing sums up the forger's logic like this: "Once my painting has been accepted and admired as a genuine Vermeer, I will confess publicly to the forgery and thus force the critics either to retract their earlier judgments of praise, thereby acknowledging their fallibility, or to recognize that I am as great an artist as Vermeer."

They did fall for it, and van Meegeren had the great pleasure of standing at the edge of a crowd and hearing one of the world's experts announce that one of his paintings was "perhaps *the* masterpiece of Jan Vermeer." And this episode greatly diminished the critics. Instead of using their expertise to assess the painting itself, they were praising it in large part because it was (they had thought) created by someone commonly agreed to be a great artist. This can be seen as embarrassing and immoral, akin to a journal editor accepting a scientific manuscript because a professor from a renowned university wrote it. From this standpoint, the psychology of how we respond to forgery has little to do with aesthetics in any real sense. It is the psychology of bias, snobbery, and prejudice.

But now consider a different view. It should not be that surprising that the responses to *The Supper at Emmaus* were affected by what the critics learned about its origin. It turns out that our understanding of history and origins is relevant to our enjoyment in every domain that one can think of. Art is not special in this respect.

For instance, the art critic Arthur Danto points out that part of sexual pleasure is surely "the belief that one is having it with the right partner or at least the right sort of partner." Same for food; part of the joy of eating is the belief that one is eating certain things: "[T]he food may turn to ashes in one's mouth the moment one discovers the belief to be false, say that it is pork if one is an Orthodox Jew, or beef, if one is a practicing Hindu, or human if one is like most of us (however good we might in fact taste)." Our pleasures are related to how we see the nature of things, and this includes their history, their origin. It matters where the meat has been—what it has touched, for instance—prior to ending up on your plate. Similarly, there are facts that one could discover about the history of a potential sex partner that could radically change one's attitude toward him or her.

Koestler draws his own parallel to sex, telling the story of a young woman in Berlin who worked for a publisher and would have sex with authors, regardless of age or gender—but only if the author's book had sold more than twenty thousand copies. She could not get sexual satisfaction from those whose works sold less. Koestler says that the woman was simply confused ("the *Kama Sutra* and the best-seller list were hopelessly mixed up in her mind"), and that we would be equally confused if we considered origin when judging artwork. But I think this is the wrong moral to draw. Koestler's example works only because the woman's criterion is so superficial— what if she instead could only get sexual satisfaction from people whom she thought of as having certain moral and intellectual qualities? Even if we were to accept Koestler's premise that all that *should* matter is the sensory event itself shorn of history, this is not how pleasure works, not for sex and not for art either.

Consistent with the importance of origins, the philosopher Denis Dutton suggests that all art involves the element of *performance*, and is instinctively understood and appreciated in this way:

> Every work of art is an artifact, the product of human skills and techniques. If we see an actor or a dancer or a violinist at work, we are constantly conscious of human agency. Less immediately apparent is the element of a performance in a painting that has hung perhaps for generations in a museum, or a long-familiar musical composition. Yet we are no less in such cases confronted with the results of human agency. As performances, works of art represent the ways in which artists solve problems, overcome obstacles, make do with available materials. The ultimate product is designed for our contemplation, as an object of particular interest in its own right, perhaps in isolation from other art objects or from the activity of the artist. But this isolation which frequently characterizes our mode of attention to aesthetic objects ought not to blind us to a fact we may take for granted: that the work of art has a human origin, and must be understood as such.

From this art-as-performance standpoint, the Dutch critics were not guilty of snobbery or magical thought when their judgments about *The Supper at Emmaus* changed. They were being perfectly reasonable. They had discovered that it was no longer the product of a creative artist with a distinct style, but a mere imitation of another's work. This mattered to them, reasonably so.

If you are not convinced, consider a movie called *Psycho*. It is about a woman who steals money from her employer and leaves town to meet her lover. Caught in a storm, she spends the night at the Bates Motel, where she meets Norman Bates, a quiet man with an unusual relationship with his mother. She is later murdered, stabbed in the shower. When this movie came out it did poorly at the box office and was described by critics as plodding and unimaginative. Nobody ever viewed it as a classic or important film.

I am speaking of the 1998 version of *Psycho,* directed by Gus Van Sant. This was a "shot-by-shot" remake of Alfred Hitchcock's classic 1960 film. Audiences who saw the movie knew it was a remake, and they knew that Van Sant knew. This affected their aesthetic responses. If Hitchcock had never made the original film, the 1998 *Psycho* would have been received in a different way. Is this really irrational?

Some would argue that a focus on an artwork's origin is not a human universal. In his discussion of artistic crimes, Anthony Julius, a lawyer, explicitly states that forgery is not a "natural" crime, because it derives from "historically specific notions" of authorship. It is sometimes said that people in some societies just don't care about where an artwork comes from.

It would help to know what young children think about forgeries. Do they value them less? We know from the studies described earlier that origins matter for how children name and categorize an artwork, but we do not know whether origins matter for how much children *like* an artwork. The closest anyone has come to exploring this question is a study by the psychologists Carl Johnson and Melanie Jacobs that found that four-year-olds understood that it would be appropriate to put the sweater of a famous person into a museum, but not an exact duplicate. This is intriguing, but a sweater is not an artwork, and the sort of history here involves personal contact, not intentional creation.

When the proper studies are done, I expect we will find that even young children take history, and particularly intentional history, seriously when evaluating art, not just when naming and categorizing it. This is because an artwork is the product of thoughtful human activity, and therefore is understood and appreciated through the same intentional interpretation that we apply to other artifacts.

THE PLEASURES OF DUALISM

We still have not fully explained why some of us *like* anxious objects.

In appreciation of these artworks all of the ingredients of pleasure discussed earlier come into play, but there is at least one more that we have not yet discussed: we enjoy displays of skill, of virtuosity, both physical and intellectual. This type of pleasure is not limited to art; it also extends to our enjoyment of athletics. In both cases, our appreciation of the finished product is contingent on certain assumptions about its origin. For art, the factor we have been focusing on so far is our inference of a genuinely creative process, as opposed to (mere) imitation, but there are other considerations as well. Dutton points out that a music lover might be awed by the speed of the double-jumps in a recorded performance of Liszt's "Mephisto Waltz"—but it would surely make a difference if she knew that this improved performance had resulted from the efforts of a skilled recording engineer. Or consider the angry reaction when the members of Milli Vanilli were caught lip-synching during a 1989 concert (their record skipped). By the same token, finishing the New York City Marathon in under two and a half hours is an admirable physical feat, but it is somewhat less impressive if the runner has been using performance-enhancing drugs, and a lot less impressive if she is discovered to have taken the subway.

Certainly not everyone enjoys the sorts of artworks discussed throughout this chapter. How impressed a person is with the act of creating these things is an important factor in their level of appreciation. Someone who admires the work of Jackson Pollock is likely to be moved by the performance that led to the origin of these paintings, and to see it as impressive and difficult. One appreciative critic starts his description of Pollock's painting *One (Number 31, 1950)* by noting that it is 9 feet high and 17 feet wide, and he goes on to review the problems of creating arcs of paint that extend over two or three feet, the difficulty of laying lines on top of each other, allowing the canvas to show through while at the same time maintaining the identity of each element, dealing with the demands of drying paint, and so on. He suggests that anyone who looks at this painting and says, "A child can do it!" should feel welcome to try it himself.

It was said earlier that we react to pictures of a scene as we would react to the actual scene. A representation of an unpleasant scene is unpleasant; a representation of something that we would enjoy seeing is pleasurable. There is a rough sense in which this is true, but it is not quite accurate. As Aristotle wrote in the *Poetics,* "The sight of certain things gives us pain but we enjoy looking at the most exact imitations of them, whether the forms of animals which we greatly despise or of corpses." I once spent an enjoyable hour in Madrid admiring Goya's spectacular painting *Saturn Devouring His Son,* but if I saw something like that in real life, I would run like hell.

An adequate theory of the psychology of art needs to acknowledge that there are two ways to look at any human creation, including artwork. This corresponds to the two ways of seeing the world we possess more generally—in terms of physical bodies and in terms of desires and intentions.

One can see art in the literal sense of *seeing,* where one responds to its perceptible properties—a natural and inevitable mode of interpretation. Because of this, we do tend to like pictures of pretty things, and react poorly to scenes of horror. It can be hard to override this primitive tendency; not everyone likes pictures of corpses. We tend, instinctively and to some extent uncontrollably, to react to a realistic picture as we would react to the actual object or scene that the picture depicts.

But we can also see art as art. When we do this we see it in terms of the performance that has given rise to its existence; we attempt to reconstruct its history, including the intentions of the artist. This determines the name we call it and the category we place it in, and it also partially determines our aesthetic reaction, sometimes overriding our more primitive mode of seeing the object as a mere object. And so a picture of an ugly thing can be beautiful, a grotesque scene of violence can be a pleasure to behold, and the most unlikely material objects can spur certain intense emotional reactions. Sometimes they can even make us cry.

PART III

THE SOCIAL REALM

4

GOOD AND EVIL

The soul selects her own society
Then shuts the door.

—Emily Dickinson

"I'll get you my pretty. And your little dog, too."

—The Wicked Witch of the West

WITH THE NOTABLE exception of lust, my son Zachary had committed each of the seven deadly sins before his fourth birthday. This is reassuring. These sins show that he is human, neither saint nor chimp. They also show that he is pretty smart. The need for intelligence is most obvious for sins that involve comparing oneself to others, such as pride and envy. But even corporeal transgressions such as greed, sloth, anger, and gluttony reflect a deliberative ranking of priorities. Both a person and a goldfish might eat too much, but only the person can be a glutton because only the person could know what he was doing and could have chosen to do otherwise.

Zachary's sins show that he is a moral creature, with the potential to willingly do right and wrong. A typical three-year-old can feel embarrassment, guilt, and shame, can become angry when treated unfairly, and, most important, can sympathize with others in pain and act to make their pain go away.

I suggest that the roots of morality are innate. They lie at the core of our evolved ability to deal with other people, a central part of our appreciation of souls. From this perspective, our moral feelings are no less adaptations than our taste for sweet foods and our perception of solid objects. Some of these moral capacities are shared with other species, but no other animal has the moral powers of a human three-year-old.

SEARCHING FOR DR. EVIL

Are you evil? I doubt it. Nobody sees himself as the bad guy. The villain of *Austin Powers' International Man of Mystery* is called Dr. Evil, but this is parody; real villains are not so self-aware.

Consider the famous threat made by the Wicked Witch of the West in *The Wizard of Oz*. It sounds sinister, but consider the circumstances. The witch's sister lies dead only a few feet away, crushed by Dorothy's flying house, and it certainly looks as if Dorothy was responsible for her gruesome demise. Seeking out vengeance for the murder of a close family member is a natural response, some would even say a moral one, especially in a lawless society such as the Land of Oz. While the filmmakers sway us away from having sympathy for the Wicked Witch of the West (starting with the ludicrous name), the story works so well in part because the witch has a plausible motivation for her rage. If someone had just murdered your sister, how would you respond?

In the real world, evildoers see themselves as good people doing good things or good people forced to do difficult things because of special circumstances, or, at worst, good people who are forced, tricked, or goaded into doing bad things, against the grain of their fine characters. The psychologist Roy Baumeister notes that people prosecuted for war crimes usually claim that they themselves are the victims. Nazi war criminals complained that they were the targets of overzealous and unfair prosecution; many of the Serbs accused of mass murder and systematic rape in the 1990s saw themselves as the injured parties, who were being blamed for carrying out just reprisals for atrocities committed against their own families and neighbors.

We can dismiss some of this as a coldhearted tactic to win sympathy or lenience, but it sometimes appears heartfelt. The gangster Al Capone once complained, "I have spent the best years of my life giving people the lighter pleasures, helping them have a good time, and all I get is abuse, the existence of a hunted man." The serial killer John Wayne Gacy, who killed at least 33 people, mostly children, would tell people that he was made "a scapegoat," and he wondered whether anyone could really appreciate "how badly it hurt to be John Wayne Gacy." A theme in more mundane day-to-day assaults is that the violence is a just reprisal—either because of what the victims themselves had done or because of what other members of their race, class, or sex had done. *They had it coming.*

Few of us see evil as an option on a par with good, a fork in the road that is willingly and knowingly traveled. The evil we commit is inadvertent, justified in the face of limited alternatives, or the result of exceptional circumstances. Some philosophers and theologians go further and argue that it is impossible to rationally choose sin. This is a theme that runs through Augustine's *Confessions,* starting with the question of why Adam, who was not deceived by the serpent, ate from the forbidden tree. Not because he chose to be evil, argues Augustine, but because he did not want to disappoint Eve, to abandon her in her terribly risky choice. As Garry Wills puts it, original sin was born of misplaced gallantry. Similarly, Augustine justified his own youthful misadventures—

stealing pears from an orchard—as the consequence of desire for companionship, a more positive motivation than coveting another's property.

Psychopaths are exceptions to the universality of good intentions. These men—they are almost always men—are not stupid or ignorant; they can understand the consequences of their actions. But this knowledge does not sway them; they lack the normal pull of conscience and feel little remorse for their actions. They do not possess moral feelings, at least not to the same extent as the rest of us. They do bad things, and they know it. As the serial killer Gary Gilmore put it, "I was always capable of murder. . . . I can become totally devoid of feelings of others, unemotional. I know I'm doing something grossly fucking wrong. I can still go ahead and do it."

Another serial killer, Kenny Bianchi, when asked what it was like to kidnap, torture, and kill young women, said, "It's like a kid going down the street and you see all these candy stores and you can pick any candy you want and you don't have to pay for it and you just take it. You just do what you want. It's the greatest."

After being captured, the serial killer Ted Bundy was puzzled about all the fuss surrounding murder: "I mean, there are so many people."

Psychopathy is treated as a mental illness—in fact, the proper clinical designation is "antisocial personality disorder," though I will continue to use the more colloquial term. It is an odd illness, different from depression, schizophrenia, and the like, because we hope to treat psychopaths not because of their own misery but because of the misery they cause others. At the same time, however, many psychopaths, such as Gilmore and company, are not successful people, even by their own amoral standards. They tend to do poorly, dying young or ending up in prison. Often they kill themselves.

Nobody knows what makes a psychopath. The disorder shows itself early; as children, psychopaths torture small animals, lie incessantly, and show little compassion or empathy. There is some heritability for just about any human trait (height, intelligence, happiness, and so on), and we know that there is a genetic component to normal children's ability to care about the pain and happiness of others. Psychopaths might be those born with the short end of the moral stick. Experience might count as well: In some experiments done in the 1950s, psychologists isolated baby monkeys from their peers and mothers for the first year of life. These babies grew to be aggressive and insensitive to the plight of others: monkey psychopaths.

In the real world, children of psychopaths typically suffer from a double whammy: they share whatever genetic propensity their parents have toward psychopathy, and they also have the bad luck of being raised by psychopaths, who, as you might imagine, are not the world's most caring parents.

NICE GUYS FINISH FIRST

The existence of psychopathy raises the question of why moral feelings exist at all. Why aren't we all psychopaths?

One can try to answer this question with an appeal to divine origins—we are said to be created in God's image, after all—or to the civilizing forces of culture and government, an answer favored by scholars with as little else in common as Hobbes and Freud. But, perhaps surprisingly, a lot of the answer comes from our animal nature.

People who do terrible things are sometimes called "animals." This is unfair to animals. Nonhuman animals are pretty nice sometimes. They display *altruism,* which among biologists means that they act in ways that benefit others at their own expense.

The most basic form of altruism is when an animal helps out its children. From a Darwinian perspective, this is a no-brainer, particularly when we keep in mind that the force behind natural selection is not increased success at survival; it is increased success at *reproduction*. Imagine, then, two animals, otherwise identical, where only one is predisposed to care for its children in a way that increases their chances of survival. Whatever heritable properties cause this animal to be a caring parent will spread through the population, because the offspring of that animal will have a greater chance of surviving and will also tend to possess these properties. Over the course of generations, all members of the population will come to possess this trait. This is the logic of natural selection: if there is variation in some trait, and this trait is passed from parent to child, the variant that leads to more offspring will tend to win out. Natural selection guarantees that animals evolve in such a way as to ensure the survival and further reproduction of their offspring, and ensures that they will grow to be, in the biologists' technical sense, altruistic, helping others at their own expense.

Animal altruism extends to other relatives as well. One way to explain this is by means of the theory of "kin selection," developed by the biologist William Hamilton and clarified by Richard Dawkins. Just for the moment, ignore the animals themselves and consider evolution from the gene's point of view. The genes that survive are those that make the most copies of themselves. But genes do not directly copy themselves; they must create biological entities such as animals, plants, and viruses to do it for them. These entities, or "vehicles," copy the genes either through asexual reproduction—cloning—or, more commonly, through sexual combination with other vehicles. Natural selection works on the genes to create increasingly better vehicles, and the success or failure of a gene depends on the prospects of the vehicle it creates. It used to be said that a chicken is merely the egg's way of making another egg; the modern variant is that an animal is merely the gene's way of making another gene.

To see the implications of this sort of shift in perspective, consider the question of why we sneeze and cough when we have a cold. From the perspective of the whole animal, these actions are merely accidental by-products of the virus. But Dawkins points out that taking the virus's point of view generates a better answer. The virus has evolved to manipulate the respiratory system of its host to expel it into the air, which then makes it more likely that other people will get infected—from the virus's viewpoint, it has found more hosts. From the standpoint of the virus—or more precisely, the standpoint of the genes that create the virus—people are merely vehicles through which reproduction takes place. One could imagine a better-adapted cold virus that infects its host's nervous system and compels the host to kiss other people on the mouth. In fact, this is pretty much the effect of the rabies virus, which motivates dogs to wander away from home, foam at the mouth, and bite other animals. Viruses are the original body snatchers.

From this genetic perspective, there is nothing special about being nicer to your children than to any other kin. For any gene, there is a 50 percent chance that it will find itself in an offspring (it is 100 percent for creatures that reproduce by cloning), but there is also a 50 percent chance that the same gene will be present in a sibling, and a 12 percent chance that it will be present in a first cousin. Successful genes will create vehicles that are altruistic toward different kin in degrees that reflect the chance of the kin sharing genes. An animal that devotes its energy equally to its child (50 percent) and its cousin (12 percent) would in the long run be worse off than one that favored the child over the cousin by a factor of about four (50 divided by 12).

In fact, there is nothing special about being nice to *yourself*; there is no reason for genes to construct vehicles that treat themselves as having a qualitatively different status from other vehicles. Imagine two animals, one that always favors its own survival, regardless of the situation, and another that would sacrifice its life for three of its children. The genes of the second animal, not the first, are likely to be sustained in a population. When the biologist J. B. S. Haldane was asked whether he would lay down his life for his brother, he reportedly did some quick calculations and said that he would not, but he would gladly give his life for three brothers, or five nephews, or nine first cousins.

Steven Pinker points out the irony in all this. This gene-centric view has been dubbed the theory of the "selfish gene" by Richard Dawkins, a label that has led to a cluster of misunderstandings, such as that our genes make us selfish or that selfishness is adaptive. But this is backward. To say that genes are selfish implies that they exist only to create copies of themselves; in a metaphorical sense, they do not care about anything else. This means that the vehicles that genes create—such as animals—are *not* necessarily selfish. To the extent that evolution occurs at the level of the genes, there is no hard-and-fast distinction between oneself and another, no categorical difference between an animal protecting itself from a predator and protecting its children or siblings. From a genetic perspective, my three brothers really are worth more than I am, and it makes perfect sense for evolution to favor the emergence of brains that guide animals to act on this fact. The generosity of animals can be the direct result of the selfishness of genes.

Altruism extends toward nonrelatives as well. Animals take great risks to warn others. Blackbirds and thrushes give warning cries when hawks are above, which gives other birds a chance to escape, at the cost of calling attention to themselves. Vampire bats, when they have the opportunity to fill up with blood from a large mammal such as a cow, horse, or person, return to the cave and kindly vomit the excess blood into the mouths of all the other vampire bats. Chimpanzees lead one another to food-laden trees and share food that they have hunted. Animals groom one another for parasites, they watch over each other's offspring, and they often withdraw during combat, choosing not to kill a defeated and vulnerable adversary. All of this altruism extends toward members of the group that are not blood relatives.

Just as an aside, many people, particularly pet owners, believe that animals' sympathy extends to those humans who care for them. For instance, the primatologist Barbara Smuts says that when she is depressed, her dog Safi "approaches, looks into my eyes, and presses her forehead against mine. Then, without fail, she lies down besides me, maximizing contact between her body and mine. . . . As soon as I am supine, she rests her chin on my chest, right on top of my heart, and locks her gaze with mine until my mood shifts." I am unsure what to make of such anecdotes, but it would be unreasonable to dismiss them out of hand. One does wonder how the animal sees the human. As a relative? Perhaps as a surrogate parent of a sort? As a member of the same tribe?

In the early days of evolutionary theory, kindness of animals toward non-kin was an embarrassment. Darwin argued that it was an absolute prediction of his theory that there could exist no structures or behaviors that are disadvantageous to an organism's survival and reproduction. If you found a horse that evolved a saddle for the pleasure of its riders, it would be devastating for the theory of natural selection. But this seems to be exactly what happens in these examples of altruism: an animal instinctively engages in a costly act for no apparent benefit to itself.

The problem of explaining altruistic acts might look as if it has an easy solution: Although it may not be adaptive for an individual animal to risk its life with a warning cry, it is adaptive for the group that the animal belongs to, since the overall benefit of everyone being warned outweighs the cost to the individual. These traits evolve because they are for the good of the group, not the individuals.

This is a tempting explanation, and Darwin himself was tempted by it, once arguing that human morality evolved because of the advantages that it gave to tribes of people, not to individuals. But evolution cannot work this way. To see why, imagine a mutant psycho-bat that takes blood from others but doesn't give any blood away; it just regurgitates the excess. Similarly, you can imagine two squirrels, a standard one that both attends to warnings from others and gives out these warnings, and a psycho-squirrel, one that attends to warnings, but never takes the risk of producing one. In the language of evolutionary theory, such mutants are "cheaters"—they take the benefits without paying the costs. They will do better at surviving and having offspring, and the genes that lead to their selfish nature will soon flood the population. The nice guys will go extinct. The harmonious and mutually beneficial social structure of warning and sharing is not, to use the term favored by biologists, an evolutionarily stable strategy. This is why the existence of altruism was such a headache for the early Darwinians.

The way out of this mess is the modern theory of reciprocal altruism. Suppose the nice guys—those with the genes for caring and sharing—paid close attention to the other members of their group so as to ensure that everyone else was just as nice. Suppose as well they were able to identify any cheating mutants and could later retaliate against them. Any mutation that led to the emergence of a psycho-gene would be weeded out. Under those assumptions, cheaters would not prosper, and altruism could flourish.

This demands a lot from an animal, though. It has to live in stable groups, and must be able to recognize distinct individuals, monitor these individuals' behavior, keep track of the cheaters, and adjust its own behaviors later on so as to punish them. Not all creatures have the cognitive abilities to do all this and not all creatures find themselves in situations where an individual can get an overall benefit by accepting an occasional cost. But some animals, including humans, plainly do.

THE MORAL EMOTIONS

Some of the altruism we have been discussing is expressed in physiological traits such the mammary glands of mammals, pouches in kangaroos, and all the other various paraphernalia devoted to the care and feeding of young. Altruistic traits might also be less obvious. For a group of lions chewing on a kill, it might be adaptive, particularly if they are close kin, for them to restrain themselves and not entirely fill their bellies, so that everyone can get the minimum amount necessary for survival. You might think that such restraint would require a complicated mental system that monitors other lions' intake of food and responds accordingly. But Dawkins points out that a much simpler mutation could do the trick—one that leads to bad teeth, thereby slowing down a hungry lion. A propensity for bad teeth could thus be an altruistic adaptation.

This is a pleasantly perverse account, but I am interested here in cases where the altruism of the biologist looks pretty much like the altruism of the psychologist and the theologian. I am interested in how natural selection might make us altruistic by shaping our mental life in certain ways, so that we genuinely care about others and will sacrifice for them. This is not the sort of analytic understanding of other minds that was discussed in the last few chapters—it is not mindreading in the strict cognitive sense. Instead it is about the drives, motivations, desires, and appetites that motivate altruistic action. We can describe these mental states as the moral emotions.

An adaptive perspective on emotions might come as a surprise. For a long time philosophers viewed emotions as nothing but trouble. Kant, and before him Plato, saw them as corrupting influences and were convinced that rational and moral behavior is driven by *reason*. The emotions are partial—they play favorites. And if there is anything that all moral theorists agree on, it is that moral deliberation should be fair.

This negative view of emotions shows up in the legal realm. In the United States, judges explicitly warn juries not to be swayed by their emotions when making judgments. In a case concerning jury instruction for sentencing, Justice Sandra Day O'Connor was explicit about the dichotomy between morality and emotions, arguing that a sentence should "reflect a reasoned *moral* response to the defendant's background, character, and crime rather than mere sympathy or emotion." A sentence should reflect a "moral inquiry," not an "emotional response."

This view of emotions also shows up in the ultimate measure of popular culture, *Star Trek*. Mr. Spock is a Vulcan, a descendant of a once-aggressive race that avoided destruction only because they learned to suppress their emotions. Vulcans live according to the cold dictates of logic. Data is a robot driven only by reason; his programming does not include emotions. Spock and Data are high-ranking officers who are respected and highly competent. Their lack of emotion gives them advantages over the more volatile humans; they do not panic, lose their temper, or fall prey to lust or pride.

But, as Pinker points out, Spock "must have had some desires and motivations. Something must have impelled him to explore strange new worlds, to seek out new civilizations, and to boldly go where no man had gone before." Spock wore clothes. When attacked, he fought or retreated; he defended his shipmates, even at risk to himself; he obeyed orders; he immersed himself in scientific problems; and he would engage in sharp debate with his shipmates. What are the motivations for these acts if not modesty, fear, anger, loyalty, curiosity, and pride? Similarly, the philosopher Richard Hanley notes that Data, over the course of just a few episodes of the television series, clearly feels regret, trust, gratitude, envy, disappointment, relief, bemusement, wistfulness, pride, curiosity, and stubbornness.

When people say that Spock and Data lack emotions, they are referring to their expressionless faces and modulated voices; they do not laugh, shout, groan, snort, snicker, pout, leer, strut, bluster or glare. But they surely have emotions. Emotions enable us to set goals and rank priorities. If we were ever to build a robot with any capacities whatsoever, let alone one that could survive and reproduce in a hostile world, it would need emotions.

The ultimate test of this claim would be to find people who have no emotions and see how they fare. Nobody like this exists. But as a rough approximation, we can look at some unfortunate individuals who suffer damage to the prefrontal cortex, which leads to a blunting of certain emotional responses.

The neuroscientist Antonio Damasio discusses the famous case of a construction foreman, Phineas Gage, who in the 1840s had an iron bar plunge through his head. In some sense, Gage was lucky; his ability to move was not impaired, his senses were mostly intact, and so were his memory and his language. But after the accident, his friends observed, "Gage was no longer Gage." He had once been an energetic and conscientious friend and businessman; now he was irreverent and profane, drinking and brawling, and could no longer hold a job. He died in obscurity.

Damasio tells of a modern Gage, a man named Elliot who had a brain tumor in the frontal lobes. The tumor was removed but the damage had been done. Elliot remained an intelligent and charming man, but "Elliot was no longer Elliot. . . . He needed prompting to get started in the morning and go to work. Once at work he was unable to manage his time properly; he could not be trusted with a schedule." Damasio blames these failings on Elliot's loss of emotions: "[T]he cold-bloodedness of Elliot's reasoning prevented him from assigning different values to different options, and made his decision-making landscape hopelessly flat."

I am proposing here that emotions, including the moral emotions, are good for you. But the existence of psychopaths poses a problem for this theory. They suffer from a deficit in moral emotions, and they succeed in life because they fake it—fake love, fake loyalty, and fake empathy, while cold-bloodedly plotting for their own benefit.

Surely compassion, guilt, and a sense of fairness cannot be all that important if psychopaths thrive without them.

Most of what we know about psychopaths is from those who get caught, or who are referred to therapy—the unsuccessful psychopaths. It is sometimes speculated that these are an atypical group. Many believe that certain phenomenally successful businesspeople and politicians are unencumbered by a conscience. You may feel an ominous twinge at the idea of smiling leaders being cold-blooded monsters, and it is not unusual to find pop diagnoses of psychopathy for presidents and other famous figures.

But the successful psychopath may be a myth. An analogy is with people who are born without the ability to feel physical pain. You might imagine this to be a wonderful state, but people with this condition are usually dead by the age of thirty. They burn themselves; they damage their joints by bending their arms and legs too far. Mere sensation and rational desire are not enough to protect the body; you need the motivating unpleasantness of actually being hurt.

The situation might be the same with psychopaths. I do not want to fetishize emotions, but they have evolved with our long-term interests in mind. A normal person's behavior is shaped by love, guilt, shame, empathy, and the like. The psychopath lacks these moral emotions, but has to live his life as if he did possess them—as if he cared for other people, as if he felt guilty after doing something bad. Without the outward appearance of some moral sense, nobody would go near such a person.

It is emblematic of the psychopath, I think, that he can be very successful in the short term, such as a one-off con game, but fails in the long term. This might be due to an inability to consciously make the same choices that someone with appropriate moral emotions does instinctively. Or it might just be difficult to motivate oneself to comply with moral rules that have no real emotive pull. (It must be *hard* to be a psychopath—so much effort, all the time.) In addition, the moral understanding of psychopaths may be somewhat impaired; perhaps they are not really as smart as they look when it comes to morality. The psychologist James Blair has argued that psychopaths lack a normal appreciation of the distinction between transgressions of social conventions, such as a boy wearing a skirt, and transgressions of the moral code, such as a child hitting another child. Normal adults and children treat moral transgressions as worse, while psychopaths do not. This might be because an appreciation of this distinction rests in part on a distinctive visceral response to the moral transgressions, a response that the psychopaths lack. But regardless of the source of their problems, psychopaths do not prosper. Nice guys finish first.

MORALITY 101:
EMPATHY AND COMPASSION

If you experience the pain and pleasure of others while maintaining the distinction between yourself and the other, you have empathetic awareness. You are on your way to becoming a moral animal.

A full-blown moral sense extends beyond this basis. We can behave in a moral fashion toward those we have no empathy for. For instance, we can work to alleviate starvation in a faraway land even if we do not in any way experience the pain of those who are starving. And there are moral notions that do not have much to do with empathy, at least not directly, such as the virtues of thrift and celibacy, or an abstract understanding of fairness and justice. There are even cases in which morality conflicts with empathy: a police officer should arrest someone for a crime even if this makes that person miserable, and even if the person's misery causes the police officer to experience empathetic distress. Still, the argument I wish to make—following many others, including contemporary philosophers such as Martha Nussbaum and developmental psychologists such as Martin Hoffman and Jerome Kagan—is that empathy is the foundation for all that follows. As the poet Shelley wrote, "The great secret of morals is love."

Empathy comes early and easily. Babies will cry at the sound of other babies crying. Non-humans have similar responses: it is torture to expose rats to the pain of other rats. In one study in the 1950s (which might now be viewed as unethical) rats were trained to press a lever for food. Then the experimenter changed the setup so that the lever sometimes provided food but also shocked another rat that could be seen in another chamber. Rats would choose to eat less (though they would not choose to starve to death) so as to avoid hurting other members of their species. Later experiments with monkeys found that they would forgo food for even longer. Their sensitivity applied only to members of their own species—they had no qualms about shocking a rabbit in order to receive food.

Why is it upsetting to see certain others being harmed? In part it is because we feel their pain—literally. Psychologists and philosophers have long observed what they term "emotional contagion"—the transmission of emotional experience from one person to another. Adam Smith in 1759 gave a simple example of this: "When we see a stroke aimed, and just ready to fall upon the leg or arm of another person, we naturally shrink and draw back our own leg or our arm, and when it does fall, we feel it in some measure, and are hurt by it as well as the sufferer."

In their fascinating book on this topic, Elaine Hatfield, John Cacioppo, and Richard Rapson posit that emotional contagion is a process characterized by two steps:

Step 1: Imitation. We imitate people, mimicking their responses and moving our bodies in anticipation of how they will react. This is instinctive. If I grin at you like an idiot, pretty soon you are likely to grin back. Laughter is infectious, yawns are notoriously so, and, if the mood is right, so are tears. When we see someone with a tic or spasm, some of us have to consciously make an effort not to imitate it, and my wife, whenever she spends more than five minutes with her Texas relatives, starts to drawl. My children have great difficulty watching someone hop or dance without doing the same themselves, and can get quite dangerous if there is a martial arts movie on television.

But imitation is typically more subtle than this. Careful experimental studies find that if you observe someone arm wrestle, your own arm will twitch; if you listen to someone stutter, your lips will move in an imitative fashion, even though you might not know this is happening. Videotape analyses have found that people imitate just about everything you could imagine: expressions of pain, sadness, happiness, embarrassment, and disgust; eye-blinking; and speech pitch and speech volume. People respond to the movements of another blindingly fast, with a lag of about one fiftieth of a second.

Some recent research has tried to pinpoint where this process takes place in the brain. When a person performs an action, such as grasping some food, certain neurons in the cortex fire, including some known as "mirror" neurons. The mirror neurons also fire if the person observes another person performing the same action. This suggests that there are parts of the brain that do not distinguish between an action that you are doing and an action that someone else is doing, which might potentially underlie our imitative abilities.

When faced with a neural system that does a remarkable task with extraordinary speed, in this case, mimicry, any biologist would immediately wonder what its purpose is. One explanation of mimicry is that it is the first step in feeling others' emotions, as part of our evolved capacity for altruism. This leads to the second part of the process.

Step 2: Changes in mood. Physical activities can have an effect on your mood; specifically, a mood-appropriate motion or action can actually cause the emotion. William James expanded this insight to a general theory of the emotions, which could be summarized as, "We feel sorry because we cry, angry because we strike, and afraid because we tremble."

The two steps come together to give us emotional contagion: by mimicking the expressions of others, we come to possess the same emotions that drove these expressions. Step 1. If you are happy, you smile; if you smile, I smile. Step 2. If I smile, I feel happy. In this way your happiness expands out of your mind and into mine.

Strange as it sounds, then, if you want people to be happy, you should get them to smile. Legions of therapists, echoing the annoying advice of parents and friends, have advised depressed people to put on a happy face, and there is some evidence that this really does work. In one study, people were asked to stick pens in the corners of their mouths either to lift their cheeks into smiles or to pull the corners of their mouths down. When shown cartoons and asked how funny they were, the "smilers" thought they were funnier than the "frowners." In another study, subjects were asked to test out different high-tech headphones. Some were instructed to listen to them while nodding, some while shaking their heads, and some while keeping their heads still. The subjects listened to an editorial arguing that tuition should be raised at their university, and were then asked their opinion of tuition raises. Those who had been told to nod tended to agree, those told to shake their heads disagreed, and those who kept their heads still were in the middle.

This analysis can go some way toward explaining why some people are so persuasive. Here is how the writer Malcolm Gladwell describes a master salesman:

> What was interesting about Tom Gau is the extent to which he seemed to be persuasive in a way quite different from the content of his words. He seems to have some kind of indefinable trait, something powerful and contagious and irresistible that goes beyond what comes out of his mouth, that makes people who meet him want to agree with him. It's energy. It's charm. It's likeability. It's all these things and yet something more.

Gladwell suggests that people like Gau are particularly gifted at manipulating the emotions of others. Nobody knows how they do this, but it might be that they tend to imitate those they interact with, and somehow a synchrony gets established. President Ronald Reagan—the "Great Communicator"—was said to be transcendently gifted in this regard. Even some people who ardently opposed him and his policies would, when watching a tape of his speech, lock on to his expressions, and would relax in sympathy when he appeared happy and tense up when he was angry.

Mimicry is hardly the only route to empathy. One can become empathetic toward someone by merely thinking about his or her plight. But mimicry might be the foundation, the special adaptation that gets morality off the ground.

How far does empathy take us toward moral behavior? Philosophers have pointed out that there is no logical reason why empathy should lead to compassion, let alone to positive moral action. Suppose you observe someone in pain and, being empathetic, feel pain yourself. Why should this lead you to care about the person in pain, to feel compassion?

Indeed, not everyone does feel compassion. Consider the response of a woman near the death camps in Nazi Germany who saw people taking several hours to die after being shot. She was sufficiently upset to write a stern letter: "One is often an unwilling witness to such outrages. I am anyway sickly and such a sight makes such a demand on my nerves that in the long run I cannot bear this. I request that it be arranged that such inhuman deeds be discontinued, or else be done where one does not see it."

She plainly found it painful to see these people being murdered, but her response was not to help them; it was to demand that it be done elsewhere. Even otherwise moral people sometimes turn away when faced with depictions of pain and suffering in faraway lands, or when passing a beggar on a city street. Aristotle discussed certain other circumstances that would reasonably block compassion in the most moral of people—such as believing that someone's misfortune is trivial, or that it is their own fault.

There is, then, no necessary link between empathy and compassion. Nonetheless, the normal response to empathetic feeling *is* compassion. This does not follow logically; it is a fact about how minds work. Indeed, there is a rich psychological literature on empathy, and some of the results from this literature are going to strike you as obvious—but perhaps also reassuring.

Empathy is associated with good behavior toward others: people who get high empathy scores on a pencil-and-paper measure also donate more money to charity and are more likely to volunteer at homeless shelters than those who get low scores. And when you make people empathetic, often by simply asking them to take another's perspective, they are more likely to help. Indeed, the intensity of an empathetic response (as measured by heart-rate increase) corresponds to how fast someone is going to offer help. Several experiments show that empathy arises when people are exposed to the distress of others, empathy elicits helping behavior, and a person who is empathetic feels better when the person in distress is actually helped.

These are important findings about human nature. We are constituted so that in the normal course of affairs, our empathetic response to the pain of others leads to compassion, and this often leads to our helping them. Adam Smith—who was hardly naïve to the forces of self-interest, as he founded an economic theory that had selfishness at its core—insisted at the very start of *A Theory of Moral Sentiments* that the happiness of others is important to us, even though we ourselves derive no tangible benefit from it.

This makes sense from an evolutionary perspective. You would not be surprised to learn that anger often leads to aggressive action, that hunger sometimes drives people to seek out food, or that lust inspires sexual behavior. This is what these emotions are for. Similarly, emotional contagion makes it possible for us to experience empathy. And empathy exists for the role it plays in altruistic behavior.

BABY MORALITY

Mimicry emerges early. If you approach a newborn baby and stick out your tongue, the baby is likely to stick out his tongue right back. One-day-old infants synchronize their body movements with those of others, 10-week-olds imitate happiness and anger, and full-fledged imitative powers emerge by the end of the first year. Figure 4.1 shows some examples of this.

The most obvious form of emotional contagion emerges soon after birth, when babies will burst into tears just by being in the presence of other crying babies. Do babies simply associate the sound of crying with misery, just as an adult will flinch at the whine of a dentist's drill? Do they mistakenly think that they themselves are crying? We know that it is more than that. Babies will cry to recordings of other babies' cries more than to other noises, and more than to recordings of their own cries.

At the same time, this sort of response may fall short of real empathy. Perhaps, for babies, seeing or hearing the anguish of others just *hurts*. And so they seek out reassurance. A ten-month-old seeing another child in pain might look sad and cuddle her mother, because this is what she does when she herself is in distress, without necessarily understanding the origin of this distress. But by about the child's first birthday, true empathy emerges. A one-year-old will often try to help someone else by means of a soothing voice or gentle touch. This reflects an understanding that someone else's distress is distinct from the child's own, along with some appreciation of what would alleviate the distress.

Further development occurs when a child realizes that the distress of other people is not necessarily soothed by what would make the child himself happy. Martin Hoffman tells the story of a 15-month-old boy named Michael who was fighting over a toy with his friend Paul, "and Paul started to cry. Michael appeared disturbed and let go, but Paul continued to cry. Michael paused, then offered his Teddy

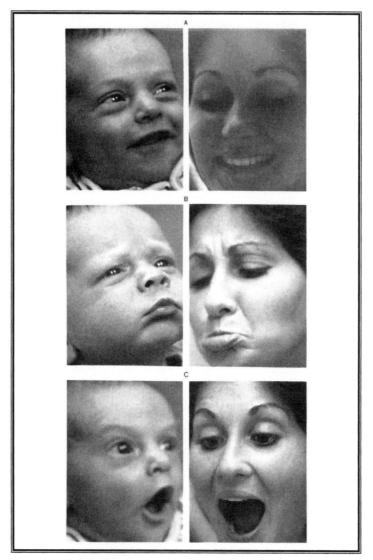

Figure 4.1 A baby mimic.

Bear to Paul. When this proved fruitless, Michael paused again. Paul finally stopped crying when Michael gave him his security blanket, which he had located in an adjoining room."

There is abundant evidence that by the time children are about two years of age, they care about others and will act to make them feel better. Both experimental and observational studies also show that children of this age often display signs of guilt after they harm someone. (As discussed in chapter 1, there are clear sex differences here—one-year-old girls are more prone to experience empathy and guilt, and more likely to help others in distress.) Babies also exhibit empathetic anger, as when a 17-month-old who sees another child receiving a painful injection cringes in pain and then smacks the doctor.

Before the child's second birthday there are some signs of embarrassment and envy—notions that require an awareness of self as a distinct and objective being. And in the following year, the child gets truly moral, being able to evaluate behavior and thought against a standard, external or internal, that gives rise to pride, shame, and guilt.

This brings us back to where we began the chapter, with a moral three-year-old. Some tantalizing studies suggest even earlier emergence of moral notions. Many investigators have observed embarrassment in children during their first year of life, as well as some behavior that looks genuinely empathetic, such as gently touching other children in distress. It might be that we are underestimating babies' empathetic capacities in their first year of life. Perhaps they do understand that others are in distress and really wish to help, but most of the time, they lack the emotional control, knowledge, and coordination to do anything. So they just burst into tears, much as an adult might respond when witnessing another person in pain but being helpless to do anything about it.

I have focused so far on the abilities of young children. But there is also an important sense in which they fall short. Young children's moral feelings lack the transcendent and universal quality that one associates with morals in a real sense.

The problem with a morality based solely on kin selection and reciprocal altruism is that it is too local. It applies only to family and friends. This is not to deny that even adults favor those with whom we share bonds of kinship and alliance. Our sense of compassion and obligations toward family and friends is almost always greater than toward strangers. But somehow we go beyond this. We come to transcend our innate, parochial, moral sense. This claim is not based on religious faith or wishful thinking. It is based on facts about humans that kin selection and reciprocal altruism do not easily explain. Human societies have legal systems and explicit moral codes. We have the capacity for kindness, and purposely do things such as giving our blood to strangers in faraway lands and abstaining from foods that we would enjoy because of concerns about the treatment of animals. We have come to adopt moral positions—the wrongness of slavery, for instance, or the notion that men and women should have equal rights—that are genuinely new to our species.

The primatologist Frans de Waal begins a perceptive discussion of morality by warning us about exaggerating the capacities of people and the differences between us and our primate relatives. Chimpanzees act as if they love their offspring, feel pain at the pain of others, and are driven to help others in need. Chimpanzees can enforce social contracts and punish cheaters, and are careful to observe and maintain social hierarchies. Nobody would doubt that such an animal has powerful social and altruistic instincts. "Animals are no moral philosophers," de Waal admits, and then asks, "But then, how many *people* are?"

This is an important question. In the next chapter, I will propose a different answer from the one that de Waal, and many others, would give: *All of us.*

5

THE MORAL CIRCLE

Article 1. All human beings are born free and equal in dignity and rights. They are endowed with reason and conscience and should act towards one another in a spirit of brotherhood.
Article 2. Everyone is entitled to all the rights and freedoms set forth in this Declaration, without distinction of any kind, such as race, color, sex, language, religion, political or other opinion, national or social origin, property, birth or other status.

Universal Declaration of Human Rights, 1948

ALL PARENTS HAVE days when they would agree with the nineteenth-century cleric the Reverend Thomas Martin when he noted the "native depravity" of children and observed that "we bring with us into the world a nature replete with evil propensities," which are "the source of all moral evil in the conduct of mankind." Or they might side with Freud, who viewed a baby as nothing more than an *id*—a polymorphously perverse bundle of desires in serious need of civilizing, first by parents, then by society. Personally, I like the way Kingsley Amis put it: "It is no wonder that people are often so horrible; after all, they started off as children."

Children really are little beasts. But perhaps being a beast is not entirely a bad thing. It is one of the oddest facts of nature that the unfeeling process of natural selection can construct creatures who themselves have feelings, who are sensitive to the pain of others, and who can work to make the pain go away.

This was the account presented in the previous chapter, and for every other species, the story ends there. But humans possess a moral understanding that transcends our innate endowment. This may well be our species' finest accomplishment, and it emerges through the interplay of our intelligence and our empathy.

SLAVES OF THE PASSIONS

Are our moral emotions, shaped by natural selection, the beginning and end of our notions of right and wrong? It certainly does not seem that way. Humans have self-control, we have language, we are conscious, we can think about the past and future, and, most of all, we can reason about morality, using our intelligence to supplement and sometimes override our evolved instincts.

At the very minimum, for example, everyone would agree that it is wrong to kill a healthy baby, sufficiently so that a society should have laws in place to forbid it. But when we deal with those who are not yet born, the issue is no longer so clear. Some believe that abortion is never acceptable. Others believe that stem-cell research should be permitted, or that abortion is acceptable in the first two trimesters but not in the third. Most people, when asked to justify their position, cite *reasons*. The fetus, even early on, is a human life and it is wrong to destroy a human. . . . The zygote is a clump of cells, nothing more, but once it grows to be viable, it becomes worthy of protection . . . Life begins at conception. . . . Life begins at birth. The psychologists Elliot Turiel and Kristin Neff have concluded that "people who differ in their views on abortion do not differ in their judgments about the value of life. Rather, they make different assumptions about when life begins."

To take a different case, the legal scholar Richard Posner argues that we are more permissive toward homosexuals and homosexual acts than we used to be just because we now know more about homosexuality. In medieval times, homosexuals were thought to be responsible for earthquakes. People used to believe that sexual orientation is a choice; now it is seen as largely genetically based and involuntary. The problem with those who discriminate against homosexuals, suggests Posner, is that they do not know any better.

This is a cheerful outlook. It suggests that as our knowledge grows, we will come to better understand moral issues such as abortion and sexual behavior. This path to moral enlightenment might be disrupted by factors such as self-interest, prejudice, and blind submission to authority, but in the end, these issues will be resolved by scientific advances and reasoned debate. The extreme version of this position was held by Immanuel Kant, who proposed that moral duty can be determined solely through a reasoning process that is autonomous from drives and emotions.

Now consider a very different perspective. Many psychologists and philosophers argue that the rational basis of moral thought is an illusion. As the philosopher David Hume famously said, "Reason is, and ought only to be, the slave of the passions." In his summary of a Darwinian theory of the evolution of morals, the writer Robert Wright claims that "our ethereal intuitions about what's right and what's wrong are weapons designed for daily, hand-to-hand combat among individuals." And the social psychologist Jonathan Haidt concludes that "moral reasoning does not cause moral judgment; rather, moral reasoning is usually a post-hoc construction, generated after a judgment has been reached."

From this perspective, the development of a moral sense is just like the development of a language. Some facts about languages are unlearned and universal, such as the existence of words and sentences; others vary across human groups and have to be learned, such as the order in which words are put together to form sentences. There is a certain period in which people are most able to learn language—if you try to learn after this period (which ends roughly at puberty), you are unlikely to speak like a native. Language learning is the product of cultural immersion, not rational choice. After all, children in Japan learn Japanese because the people around them speak the language, not because they have come to a rational decision that Japanese is better than the alternatives. In fact, all languages do an equally good job of communicating complex thoughts: the languages of Europe are not superior to those of Africa, the languages of industrial societies are not more complicated than those of isolated hunter-gatherers.

Perhaps it is the same with morality. There are universals—killing babies is wrong—and there are views particular to cultures. For many fundamentalist Christians, homosexuality is immoral and physical punishment of children is not; for many secular Americans and Europeans, it is the other way around. There is a certain period during which these culturally specific notions are best learned from parents and peers (late childhood and adolescence). And to say that one moral system is objectively superior to another is just as chauvinistic and silly as saying that one language (English? Latin? Hindi?) is superior to the rest.

This view—sometimes known as "moral relativism"—is not new. Over twenty-five hundred years ago, the Greek historian Herodotus told the story of how Darius of Persia asked some Greeks how much money he would have to pay them to eat the corpses of their fathers. They were shocked, and said that they would not do so for any price. Then, in the presence of these Greeks, Darius asked some members of an Indian tribe who *do* eat their parents' corpses how much they would take to cremate them. The Indians were horrified. Herodotus goes on to say that anyone who ridicules another's culture is "completely mad."

From this perspective, the reason why people living on the East Coast of the United States tend to favor more liberal laws on abortion than those who live in the American Midwest is not because of differences in intelligence, knowledge, or moral acumen. It is instead because certain preferences became settled in these populations in the past and are acquired by people raised within those cultures in the same way that they came to speak with certain accents and favor certain foods.

For the moral relativist, the arguments that people generate for their positions are little more than after-the-fact justifications for decisions that have already occurred. We are not like judges, considering the evidence and arguments in an objective search for the truth. We are like lawyers, trying to make a persuasive case for a preestablished point of view. People who judge that abortion is immoral in the third trimester are likely to say that they believe that the fetus is a living and experiencing being in the third trimester, and thereby worthy of protection. But it is not that the belief causes the judgment. It is the other way around.

In some cases, people flounder when asked to find reasons. Haidt and his colleagues told people about the following situation:

Julie and Mark are brother and sister. They are traveling together in France on summer vacation from college. One night they are staying alone in a cabin near the beach. They decide it would be interesting and fun if they tried making love. At the very least it would be a new experience for each of them. Julie is already taking birth control pills, but Mark uses a condom too, just to be safe. They both enjoy making love, but they decide not to do it again. They keep that night as a special secret, which makes them feel even closer to each other. What do you think about that, was it okay for them to make love?

They gave this scenario to people of different cultures, along with stories about cleaning one's toilet with a national flag, reneging on a promise made to a dead relative, having sexual relations with a dead chicken, and eating a dead dog. With the exception of some American college students at elite universities, people insisted that these were immoral acts—even though they could not articulate why, a phenomenon that Haidt calls "moral dumbfounding."

This finding illustrates a contrast between what we *think* we find immoral versus what we really find immoral. When explicitly asked, many Americans say that if an activity does not harm anyone it is not immoral and should be permitted. (Debates about the legality of prostitution and drugs often reduce to arguments over whether or not these activities are "victimless.") But when faced with certain examples where there is no harm at all, people often have the gut feeling that there is nonetheless something wrong going on.

It gets worse. The psychologist Philip Tetlock and his colleagues gave undergraduates stories in which characters contemplate certain moral trade-offs, such as a hospital administrator who must decide whether to pay for an expensive operation for a dying child. It is not surprising that undergraduates disapprove of the administrator who makes the wrong decision (refusing to pay); what is more interesting is that they also disapprove if the administrator makes the right decision (paying) *but mulls over the dilemma*. It is not enough for a person to decide to do the right thing, he must decide *quickly*. Tetlock suggests that we disapprove of people who even consider certain morally questionable options; they are tainted by the act of deliberation.

Try it out yourself. Why is it wrong to have sex with animals (but not equally wrong to eat them for pleasure)? Is it immoral for an adult to have consensual sex with a 14-year-old? (Is the answer different if we are talking about consensual heterosexual sex vs. consensual homosexual sex?) Is there a genetic explanation for racial differences in IQ? Is rape a biological adaptation? What factors motivate infanticide? What factors motivate terrorist actions, such as the attacks on the World Trade Center? Is torture ever justified? All these questions have generated angry and derisive reactions. Indeed, Tetlock's research suggests that some readers might feel a flash of disapproval toward me for writing them down, as well as some discomfort at reading them.

One unlikely victim of this sort of reaction was Descartes, whose books were banned by the Roman Catholic church soon after his death. This might seem odd, given that his books contained powerful arguments for the existence of God and the immaterial nature of the soul. But in order to make these arguments, Descartes had to take seriously these questions, to see them as topics that could be reasonably debated. This, for the church, was taboo.

I would not have spent so much time on the notion that our moral sense is not rational if I did not think there was a lot to it. We do have emotional reactions to certain situations, strong moral feelings, what Thomas Jefferson described as self-evident truths. These are not the products of rational deliberation. We just *know* that certain acts are wrong; we do not need reasons—and we are made uncomfortable when people try to find them.

At the same time, I think this view is wrong in its most central claim. Humans also possess reason and an enhanced ability to take the perspective of others. Together, these make us crucially different from other animals. As Katharine Hepburn said to Humphrey Bogart in *The African Queen*: "Nature, Mr. Allnut, is what we are put in this world to rise above."

NICE AND SMART

In many parts of contemporary secular society, talk of morals is treated with suspicion and embarrassment, and certain terms are now rarely used. When I tell people that I am interested in moral thought, a frequent reply, particularly among graduate students, is a disavowal of the concept: "I don't believe in morality" or "I don't think there really is such a thing as right and wrong." Words like "duty" and "honor" are rarely used outside a military context, and remind many people of the Klingons in *Star Trek*. When the sociologist Alan Wolfe asked a large sample of Americans what they thought of "virtue," many people had no idea what the word meant. When asked about "vice," a common reply was that it made them remember the television show *Miami Vice*.

Ironically, the absence of explicit discussion of morality is a testament to how central it is in our everyday lives. The topic is not important in the abstract because it is always important in the particular. It is like religion for the devout. And in the domain of morality, we are all devout.

Moral issues are at the core of our entertainment, including highbrow pursuits such as literature and theater and lowbrow fun like comic books and action movies. It is the focus of virtually all of our gossip—we are intensely interested in praising or condemning others, evaluating their actions and thoughts, and judging their characters and their motivations. And, protestations aside, we are all judgmental. Indeed, the ironic thing about political conservatives who worry that the humanities departments of universities are brimming with moral nihilists is that these academics are quite capable of the sharpest moral disapproval—just read what they have to say about political conservatives.

Some people are unaware they are making moral judgments—not unlike Molière's M. Jourdain, who marvels, "Good heavens! For more than forty years, I have been speaking prose without knowing it." Students who reject the language of morality have no qualms about expressing their disapproval of sexual harassment, child labor in sweatshops, and unfair treatment of graduate student teaching assistants. They are not merely saying that they themselves do not enjoy sexually harassing people and benefiting from the suffering of children and teaching assistants. They are not merely expressing preferences, like favoring wine over beer or swimming over jogging. They are saying that these are universally bad behaviors. In other words, they are saying that these acts are immoral.

From his interviews Wolfe concluded that a strong moral undercurrent runs throughout American society, even among those (such as gay men in the Castro district of San Francisco) who are explicitly permissive and nonjudgmental. Wolfe sums up the dominant philosophy in the United States as "moral freedom." This is not to be mistaken for nihilism or disinterest. Moral freedom is instead akin to religious freedom, which is not atheism, but the freedom to choose one's religion. Wolfe suggests that Americans are staunch believers in morality, but this belief is reflected in manifestly different ways. Some people might consider homosexual behavior immoral; others might find people immoral who shun others because of their sexual preference; some are appalled at those who perform abortions, others at those who block women's access to abortion clinics. "For nearly all of them," Wolfe says, "when a moral decision has to be made, they look into themselves—at their own interests, desires, needs, sensibilities, identities, and inclinations—before they choose the right course of action. . . . There is a moral majority in America. It just happens to be one that wants to make up its own mind."

Wolfe's interviewees mentioned a range of sources of moral wisdom, including self-help manuals and popular television programs; ministers, priests, and rabbis; various mental-health professionals; philosophers such as Plato and Kant; novelists such as Jane Austen and Alexander Solzhenitsyn; religious figures such as Teilhard de Chardin, the Rabbi Hillel, and Jesus Christ; and films such as *Saving Private Ryan* and *The Thin Blue Line*. In addition, Wolfe finds that the moral notions held by many Americans have been affected by three modern developments: the popularity of the language of addiction, the growing consensus that sexual preference is determined in large part through genetic factors, and an appreciation of recent developments in cognitive science and evolutionary psychology. This suggests that Posner's conclusions regarding the role of knowledge in people's judgments of homosexuality may not be as far off the mark as many social psychologists believe. Although science cannot directly tell us what is right and wrong, it can—and apparently does—inform us about background facts relevant to moral decision-making.

Some moral deliberation may be after-the-fact searches for information to help justify decisions that have already been made. But this cannot be true all of the time. In Robert Coles's descriptions of the struggles faced by black and white children in the American South during the civil rights movement, or Carol Gilligan's interviews with young women deciding whether to get an abortion, the deliberation comes first, then the action.

Also, moral deliberation sometimes drives people to act in ways that diverge from most other members of their community. Vegetarianism provides a nice illustration of this—in fact, the developmental psychologist Lawrence Kohlberg, who did the pioneering work on children's moral development, once said that his interest in morality was sparked by his own choice as a child not to eat meat. When vegetarians are asked why they choose not to eat meat, the most common reason given is ethical. Sometimes this is expressed in emotional terms—"Once my eyes were opened to the widespread sadism and torture inflicted upon farm animals, I could never eat another creature again." And sometimes it is grounded in an abstract moral principle—"In all fairness, the rights of animals to live and enjoy their lives must take precedence over our 'right' to eat whatever we desire." Most "moral vegetarians" are not raised as vegetarians and do not get their views from their schools or their religions. They are a minority in every group that they belong to. There is no powerful interest that benefits from vegetarianism, no church or corporation that profits from it. Cows have no political clout. The existence of people who hold this position shows that there is more to moral competence than simply soaking up the views of the people around you.

Admittedly, moral freedom has its limits. People do often deal with subtle and complex moral issues—debates over stem-cell research, vouchers for private schools, reparations for the descendants of American slaves—by absorbing the reactions of those who are politically and socially similar to them. Life is too short to carefully study all issues, and some appeal to authority can be reasonable, so long as the authority is legitimate. This is standard practice in science. If I need to learn something about the evolution of horses— something I know nothing about—I will check to see what experts have to say about it, and tentatively accept it as true, without demanding any other evidence. Sociologists of science have pointed out the extent to which scientific progress rests on this sort of trust, and this might hold for moral progress as well.

In any case, I have never met anyone who does not hold at least some views that are out of sync with those of the people around them. In addition, many moral issues are personal, and have to be addressed by each of us in the course of our lives: How much should I give to charity? What is the proper balance of work and family? What are my obligations to my friends? There are no off-the-shelf answers to these questions. It is up to us to decide.

MORAL PROGRESS

The twentieth century was terrible in the scope of its cruelty, including the Turkish genocide of the Armenians, the deaths of twenty million people in the Soviet Union under the Bolsheviks, the Nazi Holocaust, the Serbs' "ethnic cleansing" of the Bosnian Muslims, and the Hutu massacre of the Tutsis. There was a time when mass killings could be viewed as the responsibility of evil madmen leading people who were afraid to disobey orders. But by now it is clear that the most terrible acts are often committed by apparently normal people, as in cases when whole towns arise against some minority group, and neighbors enthusiastically kill people who used to be their friends. In light of all this, talk of moral progress might seem naïve at best.

But the twentieth century was no worse than the nineteenth, and there is clear evidence that people in modern societies are, relatively speaking, nicer to one another than we used to be. One sign of moral progress is the decrease in the incidence of murder. If you compared the per capita number of victims of homicide in modern nation-states to the figures for pre-state societies and hunter-gatherer groups, you would get the impression that we live in a heaven on Earth.

Most relevant for the purposes here is the fact that we now have moral notions different from any we have ever had in the past, and to some extent the emergence of such notions has had a positive effect on how we treat one another. This biblical command to the Hebrews is important evidence that things have changed:

> When your brother is reduced to poverty and sells himself to you, you shall not use him to work for you as a slave. . . . Such slaves as you have, male or female, shall come from the nations round about you; from them you may buy slaves. You may also buy the children of those who have settled and lodge with you and such of their family as are born in the land. These may become your property, and you may leave them to your sons after you; you may use them as slaves permanently. But your fellow-Israelites you shall not drive with ruthless severity.

Most readers, believing that slavery is wrong—people should not own other people—would now see this as an immoral command. Something else about the passage grates our modern sensibilities:

Moral codes should be universal. There should not be one law for the Israelites and another for the nations around them.

A useful way to make sense of our changing intuitions has been developed by the philosopher Peter Singer. Humans start off with instincts and emotions that have evolved through kin selection and reciprocal altruism. Since the benefits of altruism toward specific people vary, the force of our affections varies accordingly—our love for our own children is greater than for our sister's children, which is greater than for our cousins' children, and so on. Reciprocal altruism among members of a group is a parallel evolutionary phenomenon that generates a desire to help members of our group, establish bonds of trust, reward kindness, punish cheaters, and so on. But this is also graded: it is stronger toward our neighbors than to strangers. We help those who can help us. This is what Singer describes as the original moral circle.

Something has happened in the course of human history to expand this circle. We developed sympathies that extend beyond the bounds of family and tribe. We donate blood and send money to help people in faraway lands. We no longer believe that it is right to enslave the non-Israelites or their modern equivalents. Our affections extend also to animals, and to those who are disabled and retarded. As Darwin put it, something happened so that our "sympathies became more tender and widely diffused, so as to extend to the men of all races, to the imbecile, the maimed, and other useless members of society, and finally to the lower animals."

Moral progress is not sensibly viewed as akin to climbing up a ladder and kicking it away. Even as our circle expands, we still possess the original primate emotions and sentiments. These pull us toward family and friends, and away from everyone else. Social movements designed to get people to willingly dissolve boundaries between kin and non-kin—such as the traditional Israeli kibbutz, in which children were communally raised with no special bond between parent and child—have always failed. Although we may not be as biased as the Wari people of the Amazon, who describe nonmembers of the tribe with the same linguistic marker they use for food, the potential for a barbarous disregard for members of other groups lies within us. (As we will see in the next chapter, this can be triggered by emotions such as fear, anger, and disgust.)

Freud said that in difficult times, people regress to an earlier stage of development. This happens along the moral dimension when we are under threat, as in time of war or social and economic collapse. The same sort of moral regression can be induced in a laboratory. If you simply remind people in subtle ways about their mortality, they become harsher and more punitive, they identify more with their country, they like similar people more and dissimilar people less, and are more prone to disgust. Their moral circle shrinks.

But in circumstances when we are not under threat, we see glimmerings of our better selves. Consider the United Nations' Universal Declaration of Human Rights. The ideas it expresses would have been genuinely alien to people through most of human history. This is moral progress.

Does progress always lead to an expansion of the moral circle? Up until now the answer has generally been yes because our circle started off so small. But more is not always better. Is someone who believes that embryos have rights a better, more moral, person than someone who does not? Is the Buddhist who is careful not to step on an insect more morally advanced than the meat-and-potatoes man? Is Isaac Bashevis Singer right when he says that "there is only one little step from killing animals to creating gas chambers à la Hitler and concentration camps à la Stalin"? Some people might answer yes to all of these questions, but there has to be a limit. Should we demand equal rights for skin cells and personal computers? Does moral perfection require seeing a child and a rock as having equal value?

Plainly not. Some things do not deserve moral weight. To include them in the circle is not only soft-headed but unethical. Decisions within the personal, social, and legal spheres rest on trade-offs between different agents. Granting rights to fetuses limits the freedom of pregnant women, treating cows with respect restricts the pleasures of those who love the taste of meat, to refuse to experiment on stem cells means that those who suffer from certain terrible diseases are less likely to be cured. Too large a moral circle may turn out to be just as immoral as too small a one.

Things get more complicated when one considers that membership in the circle is not an all-or-nothing matter. The boundaries are vague; something might deserve only partial moral consideration, or only consideration of a certain type. The philosopher John Rawls is clear that his principles of justice do not apply to nonhumans, but he nonetheless insists that it is wrong to be cruel to them. Peter Singer argues strongly that animals should be included in the moral circle, but grants, as does everyone else, that a dog is not a chimpanzee is not a child. I imagine that very few pro-life advocates genuinely think that a zygote and a baby enjoy equal moral status, and very few pro-choice advocates believe that destroying a fetus is morally indistinguishable from tearing up a scrap of paper.

A further issue is one's obligations to others. It is likely that you believe that your children and other people's children in faraway lands are equally deserving of certain rights and freedoms, as people of equal worth. It does not necessarily follow that you have the same obligations toward all of these people. Is it immoral to spend money for your child's education instead of using the same money to rescue several other children from starvation? What about favoring the needs of your neighbors, or your fellow citizens, over those of people in distant countries? It might be that the best way to improve everyone's lot is if each person focuses most of their concern on the people around them. Or maybe this is mistaken. These are hard questions. A central aspect of moral progress is the process of working out answers to them.

IMPARTIALITY

Impartiality is the basic notion that gets moral reasoning off the ground. If I am asked to justify my actions, and I respond by saying "I wanted to" or "I can do what I please," this is not ethics. But explanations such as "It was my turn" or "It was my fair share" can be ethical, because they imply that anyone else who was in my position could have done the same. This allows justification of actions that is convincing to a neutral observer, and it makes possible standards of fairness, ethics, justice, and law.

Indeed, as Peter Singer points out, impartiality is the one thing all philosophical and religious perspectives share. It is the essence of the Golden Rule. Jesus said, "As you would that men should do to you, do ye also to them likewise." Rabbi Hillel said, "What is hateful to you do not do to your neighbor; that is the whole Torah; the rest is commentary thereof." When Confucius was asked for a single word that sums up how to live one's life, he responded, "Is not reciprocity such a word? What you do not want done to yourself, do not do to others." Immanuel Kant maintained, "Act only on that maxim through which you can at the same time will that it should become a universal law." Adam Smith appealed to an impartial spectator as the test of a moral judgment, and utilitarians argue that, in the moral realm, "each counts for one and none for more than one."

How did we come to consider impartiality so important? Singer reconstructs the development as follows: Humans started off expressing approval or disapproval with physical action, such as a caress or a slap. But when language evolved, we shifted to making verbal judgments of approval or condemnation. A judgment carries with it the notion of a standard, and can therefore be challenged. And in response to the demand for justification, a simple appeal to self-interest cannot do. Singer approvingly quotes Hume here, who notes that someone who is offering a justification has to "depart from his private and particular situation and must choose a point of view common to him with others."

A simpler version of events, though one consistent with Singer's reconstruction, is that humans come to ethics through an insight born of our powers of generalization. This was Darwin's suggestion in *The Descent of Man:* "[T]he social instincts—the prime principle of man's moral constitution—with the aid of active intellectual powers and the effects of habit, naturally lead to the golden rule, 'As ye would that men should do to you, do ye to them likewise'; and this lies at the foundation of morality."

Singer also explains how ethics can arise through reason:

> [B]y thinking about my place in the world, I am able to see that I am just one being among others, with interests and desires like others. I have a personal perspective on the world, from which my interests are at the front and center of the stage, the interests of my family and friends are close behind, and the interests of strangers are pushed to the back and sides. But reason enables me to see that others have similarly subjective perspectives, and that from "the point of view of the universe," my perspective is no more privileged than theirs.

According to this account, impartiality is not an innate idea. It is not encoded in the genes. It is a by-product of the intellect. Once a creature is smart enough, impartiality—and an appreciation of moral codes such as the Golden Rule—will emerge as a consequence of this smartness, and so all rational social beings, even those that inhabit a distant galaxy, would eventually come to develop the notion of ethics.

But impartiality only goes so far. It does not explain moral vegetarians, or those who donate their blood to people they will never know, or those who object to sexism and racism even if they themselves would profit from such arrangements. After all, the Golden Rule has been around for a long time and has been endorsed by leaders, philosophers, and theologians who saw nothing wrong with acts such as the enslavement of other humans. They were not hypocrites or fools. The Golden Rule really is compatible with slavery, so long as you restrict the moral circle so that the Golden Rule does not apply to those you would take as slaves.

To put it another way, consider again the statements, "As ye would that *men* should do to you, do ye to them likewise. . ." and "But reason enables me to see that *others* have similarly subjective perspectives, and that from 'the point of view of the universe,' my perspective is no more privileged than *theirs*" (emphasis added).

Who does Darwin include among "men"? Who is meant by Singer's "others" and "theirs"? These statements of principle do not specify. One could literally and consistently hold to the Golden Rule and believe that it applies only to—literally—men. Or one could hold that it applies to all people and also to insects and trees and computers. And so while this principle of impartiality is important—without some concept of universality you cannot have law or ethics—it does not itself explain how the moral circle might expand.

MORALITY: THE GRADUATE COURSE

Suppose you wanted to convince someone to send money to a starving child in another continent. This is not like trying to coax a hungry person to eat, or a tired person to sleep. It is not like motivating someone to come to the aid of a suffering friend or relative. Altruism toward a distant stranger is harder to initiate. It is, to use a loaded term, unnatural.

You might appeal to the intellect. After all, it is merely an accident of birth that distinguishes that distant child from a child in the person's own neighborhood or family. Ignoring the pain of people because they live far away is no more defensible than doing so because they are of a different race. (Some philosophers have called moral prioritizing according to distance "spatialism," akin to "racism.") Alternatively, you might argue that helping out the distant child will serve the broader goal of maximizing happiness, or allowing for greater fulfillment.

We might also try to generate moral action by persuading people to take the perspective of others. One example of this was President John F. Kennedy's televised speech of July 1963 in which he defended a civil rights act giving all Americans the right to equal access to public accommodations such as hotels, theaters, and restaurants. Directing his argument to whites, he did not appeal to an abstract ethical principle. Instead, he said this:

> If an American, because his skin is dark, cannot eat lunch in a restaurant open to the public, if he cannot send his children to the best public school available, if he cannot vote for the public officials who represent him, if, in short, he cannot enjoy the full and free life which all of us want, then who among us would be content to have the color of his skin changed and stand in his place? Who among us would be content with the counsels of patience and delay?

Following this, you might have better luck by getting the person to take the perspective of the child. The outcome of such perspective taking is the same that follows from the emotional contagion process discussed in the last chapter: we feel empathy.

There is no evolutionary advantage to feeling the pain of distant others. In fact, to the extent that it leads to resources being drawn from kin, it is a loss. Like our discovery of impartiality, it is an accidental by-product of other capacities. Our enhanced social intelligence allows us to reason about how other people will act and react in situations that do not yet exist, so as to plan and assess the consequences of our own actions. It is adaptive to be capable of imagining hypothetical situations and of seeing these situations from another person's point of view. And one perverse side effect of this is increased empathy. Although we have evolved to respond to actual experience—the taste of food, the smell of vomit, as well as to the sight and sound of a person in pain—we can also react to imagined circumstances. These can evoke, to a lesser degree, the same reactions as actual experience. This is what goes on when you think about food and you start to salivate and your stomach rumbles, or when you get sexually aroused at a fantasy, or break into a sweat at the thought of leaning off the ledge of a tall building. And this is what goes on when you imagine yourself in the situation of another person: you imagine the world as that person would experience it, and respond accordingly, sometimes with empathy.

Reasoned argument and emotional appeal are intimately related. Consider the influential proposal by John Rawls for constructing a just society. He proposes that, as a starting point, we imagine a group of "free and rational persons concerned to further their own interests." But the twist is that people start from a "veil of ignorance": they are constructing a society, but they do not know where they will end up in the society; they do not know their own race, sex, intelligence, class, and so on. Rawls suggests that rational people will come to agree on certain things. For purely selfish reasons, nobody would wish for a society with slavery because nobody would wish to end up as a slave. More controversially, Rawls proposes that the just society created by these rational and self-serving people would allow for differences on the basis of merit—perhaps the smarter and more motivated will end up with more money— but it will also have strong constraints as to how much inequity will be permitted.

Rawls explicitly wants to rule out the role of any sympathy or empathy here; the genius of this proposal is to generate justice through rationality and self-interest. But in a perceptive discussion, the psychologist Martin Hoffman notes that the act of practically implementing Rawls's proposal in the real world would require empathy because in fact we do not operate from a "veil of ignorance." Why would a slave owner choose to adopt the veil of ignorance? Hume famously wrote that "'tis not contrary to reason to prefer the destruction of the whole world to the scratching of my little finger." Some extra impetus to motivate people to move toward justice is needed. Hoffman suggests that empathy might provide this impetus.

Also, once the decision is made to go ahead and assume a veil of ignorance, the actual project requires considerable imaginative powers. A person has to imagine what it would be like to exist in certain circumstances. In order to conclude—from a purely self-interested stance—that slavery is wrong, the person needs to conclude that it would be unpleasant to be a slave, and this requires the ability to understand others' perspectives.

Empathy and reason also interact when it comes to the question of who falls into the moral circle. A former colleague of mine who was deeply immersed in cognitive neuroscience insisted, on the basis of current theories of brain function, that it is wrong to eat any creature with an amygdala—a structure in the brain that mediates emotion. (Those without it were fair game.) This position led him to try to see the plight of such creatures—and to avoid any temptation toward empathy for the amygdala-less. Here, reason motivates empathy. My sister Elisa is the opposite case: when she was eight years old she gave up meat because of her spontaneous empathetic concerns about the animals around her. But this empathy led her to actively search for rational arguments to support her choice.

Similarly, someone who is convinced, through rational deliberation, that slavery is wrong can then choose to take the perspective of a slave, and thereby appreciate—at a gut level—the immorality and unfairness of the situation. And someone who, for whatever reason, has taken the perspective of a slave and thereby feels empathy might be driven to explore the notion that slavery in general is immoral. Empathy and rationality can be mutually reinforcing.

The choice to take another's perspective might not be direct; we sometimes expand our moral sensibilities by controlling the situations we put ourselves in, just as a dieter may choose not to walk down the ice cream aisle of the grocery store for fear that he might succumb to temptation. Even young children, when told that they can get several cookies later on if they can hold off from grabbing a single cookie now, will consciously engage in tactics such as looking away or covering up the plate so as to distract themselves from the immediate temptation. If you believe that you *should* like members of a certain group, you can put yourself in a context that will activate more primitive positive reactions toward them, and avoid situations that reinforce prejudice. This might be something as simple as seeking out books and movies that portray such people in a positive light, and avoiding those that do not.

We also use our reasoning powers for less noble purposes. In one study, college students were told that they were going to hear an appeal for help by a homeless man, and they were given a choice—hear the man asking them to imagine what he is going through or hear him giving a simple objective appeal for help. When the students were told that if they responded to either one of the appeals they would be asked to provide a great deal of assistance, involving hours of time, they chose the objective appeal. They did not want to be tempted to imagine the man's position, because they did not want to feel empathy, and they did not want to feel empathy because they did not want to be convinced to help and then to have a large commitment. This is a laboratory analogue of turning your gaze away from a beggar because you do not want to be emotionally affected.

In the antebellum South, slave owners used their intelligence to defend slavery, arguing that, after all, a manager devotes more care to a machine that is owned than to one that is rented. They also pointed out that slavery was grounded in scripture. In Genesis, Ham viewed his father, Noah, drunk and naked and mocked him. God then condemned Ham's son Canaan and all of his descendants to be "servants unto servants." This justified the enslavement of the Canaanites by the ancient Hebrews, and eventually Americans cited the story to justify the subjugation of Africans, who, they said, were the modern descendants of Ham and Canaan.

Nazi doctors also purposefully acted so as to avoid feeling empathy for the people they were experimenting on. This distancing process included the use of euphemisms such as "transfer," "resettlement," and "selection" to blunt the reality of brutal actions. One scholar of the Holocaust has reported that he went through tens of thousands of Nazi documents, and found the word "killing" used just once—in reference to an edict concerning dogs. Some emotional distancing techniques were more extreme: the psychiatrist Robert Jay Lifton has suggested that these doctors made the choice to create a second self, a process Lifton calls "doubling"; this "Auschwitz self" allowed them thrive in the concentration camps while feeling little or no pangs of conscience.

A simpler day-to-day technique with which to thwart our better selves is to act quickly. When I break a diet, I tend to eat fast, so as to get the food into myself before I have time to think things over. The philosopher Jon Elster tells the story of how, after World War II, the Belgians realized, on the basis of experience in the previous world war, that the punishments for collaborators would be more fair and compassionate if the trials did not take place immediately. Collaborators who were tried immediately were often executed; this was less likely to occur after some time had passed and passions had cooled. For this reason the Belgians wanted the trials to proceed as quickly as possible.

FORCES OF MORAL CHANGE

We can now start to understand the puzzle of the expanding moral circle by appealing to three considerations:

Impartiality. Impartiality neither expands nor shrinks the moral circle. But once the circle exists, a grasp of the principle of impartiality allows for the formation of broader principles of justice and law, such as the Golden Rule.

The extension of empathy. We can take the perspective of those who would not naturally fall into our moral circle. Empathy can be triggered by experience, motivated through persuasion, or grounded in the application of a principle.

Formation of generalizations and explanations. We can ponder what distinguishes those within the moral circle from everyone else, and use our generalizations and explanations to motivate further perspective taking.

These notions exist in all human groups. Why then do cultures differ in their moral perspectives? How can moral change occur? Most important, why has the moral circle been expanding? We might all have become like the Nazi doctors, using our intelligence to diminish our moral circle. That the opposite has happened is due to four main factors.

1. Mutual Interdependence

Vampire bats, gazelles, and people prosper if they cooperate with other members of the species. But people are unique in that we possess the means to communicate, the intelligence to work toward beneficial agreements, and the technology to interact across great distances. In his ambitious theory of biological and cultural progress, Robert Wright suggests that such forces are driving our species to ever-increasing interdependence. Our interactions are not zero-sum, where the advantages of one individual are at the expense of another; they are win-win.

A happy consequence of this process is an increased care for others, a broadening of our moral circle. This is because of enlightened self-interest. Even if we had no preexisting moral notions, any smart creature would recognize the profit in treating others in a positive way. As Wright puts it, "One of the many reasons I don't want to bomb the Japanese is that they built my minivan."

This is reciprocal altruism writ large. At the evolutionary level, mutual interdependence benefits the genes; at the cultural level, it benefits the individuals. Selfish motives breed selfless action.

2. Contact

Hunter-gatherers lived in small groups, and for most of the life of our species, people did not go far from where they were born. But the circle of contact has been continually expanding, and the growth has increased radically over the last several decades. We find ourselves in contact with an increasing number of people.

This would be a bad thing if familiarity bred contempt. But under the right circumstances, it has the opposite effect. After World War II, the psychologist Gordon Allport proposed his "contact hypothesis": that contact reduces prejudice, particularly when the contact takes place in conditions where everyone is of equal status, they work together for a common goal, and there is social support for the contact. This theory was supported by several studies in the 1950s—white housewives who lived in desegregated public housing later had higher opinions of blacks than those who lived in segregated housing; white police officers who were assigned black partners later had fewer objections to taking orders from qualified black officers. The psychologists Thomas Pettigrew and Linda Tropp recently reviewed over two hundred studies that involved a total of over ninety thousand subjects and found overwhelming evidence for the contact hypothesis: people who spent time with members of a range of groups, including racial minorities, homosexuals, and the disabled, came to feel less prejudice toward these groups.

Research into the contact hypothesis has typically focused on situations where people have been brought together through desegregation, busing, a change in hiring practices, or some other enforced act. But some of the cases studied have been where contact was less systematic. The philosopher Jonathan Glover gives examples of cases in which chance events have led people to see the humanity of others even under the worst possible conditions. One of his examples is George Orwell: when fighting in the Spanish Civil War, Orwell came across a half-dressed enemy soldier holding up his trousers with both hands: "I did not shoot partially because of that detail about the trousers. I had come here to shoot at 'Fascists,' but a man who is holding up his trousers isn't a 'fascist'; he is visibly a fellow creature, similar to yourself, and you don't feel like shooting at him."

Similarly, a Vietnam veteran reports the discomfort that his men felt at removing belongings from dead Vietnamese and finding pictures of parents, girlfriends, wives, and children. This made them think: "They're just like us."

We sometimes try to change people's environments so as to change their morals, and this can include manipulating contact. Parents will often put their children in a certain day care or school to expose them to children of different races and different social and economic classes, with the goal of heading off prejudice, and contact-hypothesis research suggests that this is a reasonable tactic. It is similarly reasonable to put adults into group situations in which they are dependent on one another, working for a common goal, as in a sports team or military unit.

Finally, contact does not have to involve actual physical interaction. It can be presented through images and language. We can become familiar with other people through hearing stories about them, both realistic, as in the case of journalism, and imagined, as in various forms of fiction.

3. Persuasion Through Images and Stories

Sometimes the manipulation of others is more direct: a simple demand that one take the perspective of another. Indeed, many developmental psychologists see this as the driving force of moral socialization. Children are exposed to thousands of interactions where they hear sentences such as "How would you feel if someone did that to you?" This sort of nagging may have some effect: parents who use a lot of these inducements tend to have children who adopt their moral views.

Such persuasion is not limited to dealing with children: John F. Kennedy demanded that whites take the perspective of those they were discriminating against. Or consider Greek dramas; according to Martha Nussbaum, these plays

> . . . moved their spectators, in empathetic identification, from Greece to Troy, from the male world of war to the female world of the household. Although all of the future citizens who saw ancient tragedies were male, they were asked to have empathy with the sufferings not only of people whose lot might be theirs—leading citizens, generals in battle, exiles and beggars and slaves—but also with many whose lot could never be theirs—such as Trojans and Persians and Africans, such as wives and daughters and mothers.

We have known since Aristotle that we are most empathetic toward those we are familiar with and similar to, and much persuasion consists of trying to convince others that the potential targets of empathy really *are* familiar and similar. Televised or printed appeals to help starving children will inevitably include images of those children, as an attempt to elicit empathy. And language can draw us to see these individuals as if they were family or neighbors. Terms such as "brotherhood," "sisterhood," "family of man," have great evocative force. Those who wish to extend the empathy of others toward fetuses and embryos are wise to use expressions such as "preborn children" and show pictures that depict them as resembling babies; those on the other side are wise not to.

4. The Accretion of Moral Insight

In chapter 2, I discussed how children are natural scientists, trying to discover the essences of things. Similarly, Lawrence Kohlberg described children as little "moral philosophers." They are not passive recipients of moral learning; instead their moral thoughts develop in part through their own ruminations about the world. People can come to their own moral insights, deciding that it is wrong to eat meat, or keep slaves, or sit passively while people are murdered in the Holocaust.

But this capacity of individuals does not by itself explain progress. Presumably we were always moral philosophers, capable of insight and discovery, in the same sense that we were always intuitive scientists, seeking to explain patterns in the world. Moral progress occurs in part because our insights can accumulate.

The appropriate analogy here is with science. It was not I who came up with the theory of natural selection, or who discovered that the earth revolves around the sun. I learned such facts and theories from those around me, who had the advantage of those who came before them, and so on. Similarly, it was not I who figured out that slavery is a bad thing; that was something I picked up from others. In both morality and science, each generation has the advantage of the insights of all the generations that have come before.

These four factors constitute a theory of cultural development, an attempt to explain how the moral circle has come to expand over human history. But it is also a theory of individual development. Children start off with very local attachments; they resonate to the people around them, most of all to their families. This is the circle they start with. They are in this regard just like chimpanzees, monkeys, gibbons and, presumably, our shared primate ancestors. But each of the four forces described above will draw children to expand this circle. It follows that children will grow to be generous in their moral perspective if they

> . . . are brought into increased contact with other individuals.
> . . . interact with them in circumstances where cooperation leads to mutual benefit.
> . . . are exposed to stories, real and imagined, that motivate them to take the perspective of distant others.
> . . . are exposed to the moral insights of previous generations.

THE LONG VIEW

If there exist forces that drive a culture toward moral growth, analogous to forces that drive a society toward scientific growth, then what do we make of moral disagreement? The anthropologist Richard Shweder observes that people

> . . . have found it quite natural to be spontaneously appalled, outraged, indignant, proud, disgusted, guilty, and ashamed by all sorts of things: masturbation, homosexuality, sexual abstinence, polygamy, abortion, circumcision, corporal punishment, capital punishment, Islam, Christianity, Judaism, capitalism, democracy, flag burning, miniskirts, long hair, no hair, alcohol consumption, meat eating, medical inoculations, atheism, idol worship, divorce, widow marriage, arranged marriage, romantic love marriage, parents and children sleeping in the same bed, parents and children not sleeping in the same bed, women being allowed to work, women not being allowed to work.

Not all of these differences are moral ones. The hallmark of morality is the presupposition of universality: if it is wrong, then it should be wrong for everybody. In this regard, moral judgments are to be distinguished from preferences and conventions. People might be appalled at those who violate social rules and be disturbed when they themselves are out of sync—showing up at a party underdressed is a familiar example—but they can still appreciate that the rules are arbitrary, and that a different culture might do things in a different way. The psychologists Larry Nucci and Elliot Turiel found that religiously brought up children were quite clear about the distinction with regard to the precepts of their own faiths—they distinguished between rules prohibiting stealing and hitting and rules about the practice of their faith such as days of worship, head covering, kosher foods, and circumcision. They were adamant that restrictions on stealing and hitting applied to everyone, while the religious laws did not.

But some moral attitudes, including some that are grounded in religious belief, are thought to apply universally. People whose opposition to abortion is grounded in their Catholic faith are not just saying that Catholics should not have abortions; they are saying that *nobody* should have an abortion.

Moral differences persist for several reasons. For one thing, moral progress does not mean that all groups converge on the same moral system. We all live in the same physical world: electrons are the same in Holland, India, and Papua New Guinea, and so in the end, there should just be one theory of physics. But morality is more like botany. Imagine two groups separated by thousands of miles each developing its own theories of the botanical world. Each group's theory might improve, provide better description and explanation of plants, and the theories would converge with regard to the properties that all plants share. But still, the theories might end up quite different, since they have been developed to explain local phenomena. Some moral concerns are also local, dependent on certain facts about a society and its history.

Also, moral progress is *difficult*. Morality is personal in the way that most of science is not. If you tell people they are wrong in what they think about how objects move through space or why water freezes, they might be confused or irritated. But this is nothing compared to the reaction one gets when you tell them their morality is off-base and they must turn the other cheek, forgive their enemies, give up on owning slaves, accept women into the academy, not eat meat, give away most of their resources to strangers, and so on.

Finally, moral progress is difficult as well because of the connection of morals with religious beliefs. A lot of what we see as right and wrong is based on the authority of sacred texts and beliefs about the wishes of spirits and deities. These beliefs are insulated from empirical evidence and can twist morality in unpleasant ways. As a contemporary example, the self-help guru Dr. Laura recently argued that homosexuality is immoral, and cited scripture as proof. This provoked a well-circulated response over the Internet.

Dear Dr. Laura,

Thank you for doing so much to educate people regarding God's law. I have learned a great deal from you, and I try to share that knowledge with as many people as I can. When someone tries to defend the homosexual lifestyle, for example, I simply remind him that Leviticus 18:22 clearly states it to be an abomination. End of debate. I do need some advice from you, however, regarding some of the specific laws and how to best follow them.

When I burn a bull on the altar as a sacrifice, I know it creates a pleasing odor for the Lord (Leviticus 1:9). The problem is my neighbors. They claim the odor is not pleasing to them. How should I deal with this?

I would like to sell my daughter into slavery, as it suggests in Exodus 21:7. In this day and age, what would be a good price for her? . . .

Leviticus 25:44 states that I may buy slaves from the nations that are around us. A friend of mine claims that this applies to Mexicans but not Canadians. Can you clarify?

I have a neighbor who insists on working on the Sabbath. Exodus 35:3 clearly states he should be put to death. Am I morally obligated to kill him myself?

One point of this is to expose Dr. Laura as a hypocrite—she is not really objecting to homosexuality because of biblical authority; she just cites scripture to support moral intuitions that she has for other reasons. (She is hardly unusual in this practice—scripture has been used selectively to support moral positions ranging from the enlightened to the barbarous.) But the letter is also striking as an illustration of how things have changed. You can list these biblical requirements to embarrass someone, comfortable that nobody would take them seriously.

I should qualify this: almost nobody. There are places in the world in which such views are still held. But these are societies that are insulated from the processes of moral progress discussed above, relatively isolated from interaction, contact, and forms of persuasion such as books and movies. Their existence is no more of an argument against moral progress than the existence of creationists is an argument against scientific progress.

The potential for moral progress is a lucky accident. It emerges from capacities that have evolved through natural selection—including our uniquely human capacity to understand the thoughts and feelings of others. This appreciation can be enhanced and expanded, and hence the moral circle can expand. A favorite line of Martin Luther King, Jr.'s was "The arc of the moral universe is long, and it bends towards justice."

THE BODY
AND SOUL EMOTION

In Tierra del Fuego a native touched with his finger some cold
preserved meat which I was eating at our bivouac, and plainly
showed disgust at its softness; whilst I felt utter disgust at my
food being touched by a naked savage, though his hands did
not appear dirty.

—Charles Darwin,
The Expression of the Emotions in Man and Animals

Cover thy breast, it offends me.

—Molière

BABIES AND TODDLERS will happily play with, roll around in,
and even eat substances that make their parents gag. My son
Zachary, when he was two and a half years old, showed no disgust at
all, just curiosity. During diaper changes he would frequently demand, "Show me the poo-poo!" and would, if he were permitted,
scoop it up to get a closer look. Freud believed that children are very
fond of their feces—he suggested both that they see excretion as
akin to childbirth and that they view feces as substitute penises—

but I saw none of this in Zachary. He showed no sense of loss when his soiled diaper was dropped into the pail. He just saw feces as an interesting substance that appears from his body as if by magic.

Zachary's older brother, Max, was different. Max was five at that time, and his aversion to disgusting things was much like my own. If anything, he was overly fastidious. He could not bear to be present during his brother's diaper changes, and showed an almost comical aversion to urine, blood, and vomit. Max was also cautious about the contact between different foods on his plate. If a disfavored item touched some food, that food was no longer fit to eat. William Ian Miller describes in *The Anatomy of Disgust* how his own young children grew to be excessively concerned about their own bodily wastes. His daughter refused to wipe herself after going to the toilet because she was worried about sullying her hand; his son would insist on removing both his underpants and his pants if even a drop of urine went astray.

As Miller points out, disgust is a risky topic. Most writing does not take on the quality of its subject matter; one can write about boredom without being boring, or about humor without being funny. But disgust has evocative powers beyond an author's control. If you write about disgust, you are likely to end up eliciting disgust, and this is a worrying imposition to place on a reader. Also, the topic, and particularly some of the descriptions, might seem juvenile, the stuff of low comedy. Miller struggles with these concerns throughout his book, and at one point gets so worried about not being taken seriously that he abruptly cuts short a fascinating discussion of snot.

But the benefits of looking closely at disgust are well worth the risks. The study of precisely what we view as disgusting can give us insight into how our thoughts of bodies relate to our thoughts of souls. The potential to think of people and their actions as disgusting is intimately related to whether you see someone as a physical body, in which case disgust is hard to avoid, or as a soul, in which case you can transcend it. This duality of perspective has moral and political consequences in such disparate realms as genocide and sexual passion.

BAD TASTE

The word "disgust" comes from Latin and means, literally, "bad taste." And there is good reason to believe this emotion has a lot to do with food and eating. When people are disgusted, they make a certain facial expression, and this expression, as Darwin pointed out, is plainly an attempt to ward off odors, by scrunching the nostrils, and to expel unwanted food, by clenching the jaw and thrusting the tongue outward.

Also, disgust can cause nausea, which is a sensation highly relevant to food and eating. In the 1960s, the psychologist John Garcia discovered that when a rat is given a novel food and later nausea is induced by means of drugs or a high-dose of X-rays, the rat will develop an aversion to this novel food. This "Garcia effect" applies as well with humans, and can override conscious knowledge and desire. If you eat sushi for the first time and later experience nausea in connection with the flu, you might find yourself unable to stomach raw fish ever again. Even if you know full well that your nausea was caused by the flu, the very thought of sushi—its smell and taste— may inspire queasiness.

Nausea can cause vomiting. Vomit is a wonderful multipurpose substance; it is both an effect and a cause of disgust. At the same time that vomiting empties the stomach of anything you have eaten, its smell and appearance can produce nausea and thus more vomiting in yourself and others. In this way, vomit serves as a form of nonverbal communication, one that bypasses conscious reasoning. When you vomit, it is like shouting, "We may have eaten poisonous food. Everyone, stop eating, and empty your stomachs!"

Paul Rozin, a psychologist who has done much of the research on disgust, notes that there are many reasons one might avoid eating certain things without being disgusted by them. Some things are not thought of as food, such as rocks and bark. Some are deadly, like arsenic. (You would be terrified at the notion of being forced to drink tea laced with arsenic, but you would not find it disgusting. Your face wouldn't scrunch up; your bile wouldn't rise.) Some potential foods are forbidden for religious reasons, like pork for Jews and Muslims, or beef for Hindus. Some foods taste bitter, or are too bland, or too spicy. Even babies have preferences. They prefer the sweet to the bitter; if you wish to please a baby, you are better to offer sweet milk than sour pickles.

So what does elicit disgust? The best way to answer this is to look at why this emotion exists in the first place. Rozin points out that humans suffer from the "generalists' dilemma": We are not limited to a single source of food. We are not herbivores such as koalas, destined to eat only eucalyptus leaves; neither are we carnivores, like lions. We are omnivores, born into environments in which we must choose among an ever-changing array of food sources, including fruit, vegetables, and animal flesh. Agriculture, the domestication of animals, and elaborate food preparation technology have enabled modern humans to create an extraordinary universe of potential foods that no other creature would ever have dreamed of consuming, including alcoholic beverages, spicy foods, and processed cereals. But even hunter-gatherers faced the generalists' dilemma.

This world of opportunity is mostly a good thing, because when one food source is scarce, we can move to another. On the other hand, some of these foods can kill us. One hazard is plants, which have evolved chemical poisons as a defense against being eaten by herbivores. Even in urban America, many calls to poison control centers are made when children have become sick by eating houseplants.

Meat poses its own special problems. Here, the problem is the invisible microorganisms that can live within meat and multiply exponentially, resulting in contamination. You do not want to touch rotten meat, and you certainly should not eat it. You want to be as far away from it as possible. It is disgusting.

Now we can begin to understand what sorts of things elicit disgust. Nonbiological natural things like mountains and clouds are never disgusting, and neither are artifacts, with the notable exceptions of those made specifically to resemble disgusting things, such as plastic vomit. Plants are rarely disgusting by themselves, except for rotting vegetation, which is similar in appearance and touch to rotting flesh. Disgust is an emotion revolving around meat and meat by-products, substances that carry risk of disease and contagion.

BETTER SAFE THAN SORRY

Disgusting things are contaminating; any contact, however minor, is repulsive. This is not true of dangerous things in general. I might walk around with a vial of hemlock; I might keep it in my desk, nestled against my lunch. But I would not want to walk around carrying a dog turd, and if I had to, I would take pains to keep it away from my body and my food.

Various psychological experiments take this revulsion to interesting extremes. If you swish a sterilized cockroach in a glass of milk, you are not going to find anyone willing to drink the milk. Nor will anyone want milk that has been poured into a brand-new urine container, or stirred with a brand-new fly swatter. Nobody wants to eat out of a bedpan, even if it has been swabbed shiny clean. People often refuse to hold rubber vomit in their mouths, and would rather not eat fudge that has been baked in the shape of dog feces.

Irrational? After all, the subjects have been reassured that the cockroach has been sterilized, the fly swatter is new, and the bedpan is clean. Imitation vomit and fudge feces are harmless. Rozin and his colleagues note that disgust obeys the two laws of sympathetic magic that were described by the anthropologist Sir James George

Frazer in *The Golden Bough*. The first is the law of similarity, or homeopathic magic, whereby "appearance equals reality." Voodoo depends on this law. A voodoo doll resembles a person, and hence stands for it, and so stabbing the doll equals stabbing the person. The second is the law of contagion, whereby physical contact leads to the transfer of properties. Both laws arguably apply in the domain of disgust: fake feces are treated as if they are real (similarity), and if an object touches some feces, that object itself becomes disgusting (contagion). And so the experiments show that we are not rational beings; the laws of magic sway us.

Yet, at least in the domain of disgust, these biases often make sense. First, a belief in contagion is rational. Disgusting things really *are* contagious; germs really *do* transmit by contact. Maybe the nice graduate student is very responsible, and the cockroach really has been sterilized, the fly swatter is brand-new, and the bedpan has had a darn good scrubbing. But why take the chance? You don't lose anything by refusing to consume the questionable substance, after all. The moral here, as in so many of our cognitive systems, is: Better safe than sorry.

What about similarity? Even if you know that imitation dog feces are made of chocolate fudge—even if you baked it yourself, placing the fudge inside a feces-shaped mold—you might still be reluctant to take a bite. Isn't this irrational? To some extent it is, but, at worst, it is an inevitable by-product of a system that has evolved to do rational things. As discussed in chapter 2, our minds have evolved to focus on the deeper properties that objects possess—but the way we know about these deeper properties is by the information we get through our senses. And use of our senses makes us vulnerable to false alarms, cases where something looks like one thing but actually is another. Flickering images on a television screen, which we know full well to be nothing more than patterns of light on a two-dimensional array, can scare the heck out of us, make us hungry, inspire sexual passion, and cause us to sob. Our minds have evolved in a world in which it pays to take seriously what you see.

In any case, caution is a particularly good strategy when faced with a three-dimensional object. For any such object there are multiple cues to what it really is; these include what it looks like as well as what people tell you about it. Trusting your eyes, as a general rule, is wise because the surface appearance of an object is an excellent cue as to what it really is.

In the novel *Empire Falls,* Richard Russo describes a troubled teenager who tries to goad his girlfriend into taking a revolver and then putting it against her head and pulling the trigger, assuring her that there are no bullets in the cylinder: "If you knew by the evidence of your own senses that the gun wasn't loaded, then you had nothing to fear." The teenager is wrong, however; the rational act is *not* to play such a game, because the benefits of being right are so slight and the cost of being wrong is so high. The risks are much lower in the psychology experiment, of course, but the moral still holds: Better safe than sorry.

Although I am defending the rationality of disgust in general, not every disgust reaction makes sense. You can be *too* safe, after all; there are people who refuse to handle money, touch doorknobs in public places, or use toilets outside their own house. And just consider the irrationality—not to mention the immorality—of being disgusted by women, or Jews, or blacks. Although disgust might have adaptive origins, it can go seriously awry.

UNIVERSALS OF DISGUST

No discussion of the development of disgust would be complete without some mention of Freud, who lumped disgust together with shame and morality as "reaction formations," which occur to block the consummation of unconscious urges. We really *want* to eat feces, have sex with our siblings, cavort with corpses, and so on, and reaction formations such as disgust exist to block these libidinal desires.

There has to be a grain of truth here. If these behaviors were inconceivable, then there would no need for emotions to evolve (either through biological evolution or cultural development) to block them. An intuitive disgust toward drinking urine would not have emerged if it weren't that urine would otherwise fall into the range of conceivable things to drink. But this is a far cry from saying that we have *specific* desires toward the disgusting, a claim that is scarcely plausible.

A different theory derives from the work of the anthropologist Mary Douglas on pollution and taboo. She views polluting substances as those that are anomalous and do not fall into prevailing structures. Bats are disgusting, for instance, because they are freaky—they are mammals that fly, and mammals *shouldn't* fly. A person with too much body hair is disgusting because fur is a marker of nonhuman animals; missing limbs may evoke disgust because people typically have all of their limbs. But this proposal was never intended to explain disgust in general and it would do a poor job of doing so. Not all anomalies are disgusting: dolphins are mammals that swim, as freaky as those that fly, but we do not find dolphins disgusting. And consider other anomalies: a telephone baked inside a cake, a chicken sitting on the throne of a king, or a helicopter made out of peanut brittle. These are weird, but the weirdness does not inspire disgust. And the prototypical target of disgust, feces, is not at all anomalous.

Another theory roots the development of disgust in social learning. Many psychologists, influenced by Freud, believe that children's disgust about bodily waste emerges as the product of toilet training. You take a child who is initially neutral about bodily products, the story goes, and then you instill shame and humiliation over his or her messes, through angry words and horrified expressions. This is internalized, until the child's own feces and everyone else's is associated with the emotion of disgust. Same thing for blood and vomit, and for things that are considered disgusting within a particular culture, such as slugs for many North Americans.

But this is implausible for many reasons. For a start, things have changed since Freud. In my neighborhood, at least, parents don't toilet-train children by grimacing, gagging, and telling them that they are horrid creatures. Many modern parents are themselves socialized to be careful not to make their children feel ashamed by their excretion, in large part because experts in child care are staunch believers in social learning. Consider this typical example ~f *t*h*e* best child-care books around, Penelope Leach's *Your*

> *the child share your adult disgust at feces.* He just dis-
> y come out of him. He sees them as an interesting
> ng to him. If you rush to empty the potty; change
> lious fingertips and wrinkled nose; and are angry
> es or smears the contents of his potty, you will hurt
> don't have to pretend to share his pleasurable inter-

est—discovering that adults don't play with feces is part of growing up—but don't try to make him feel they are dirty and disgusting. If he knows his feces are disgusting to you, he will feel that you think he is disgusting too.

If the social-learning account of disgust were right, you would think that modern parents would have created a race of children liberated from disgust, free to touch, sniff, and devour all the objects and substances that the world has to offer.

In fact, there is no evidence that the emergence of disgust has anything to do with toilet training. Everyone is disgusted by much the same things; it does not matter whether you are raised by psychoanalysts, contemporary child-care experts, or hunter-gatherers.

A proponent of the social-learning theory might suggest that adults try to block our disgust . . . but fail. We just can't help it, our revulsion shows in subtle and unconscious ways, children pick up these cues, and learn to be disgusted themselves. But this subtle-cueing theory is not plausible. Although children have impressive abilities to understand the minds of others, they are not *literally* mindreaders, and there is no evidence that they have the power to discern such deeply hidden emotions on the part of adults. And even if they had such a power, their response to feces and the like would be way out of proportion. After all, parents get red in the face and scream at children about the dangers of licking electrical sockets and stepping off the sidewalk onto the street, and the outcome is not disgust at or fear of sockets and cars. Why then would there be such an excessive response to subtle cues during toilet training? To explain this discrepancy, you would have to say that children are born with a predisposition to grow disgusted by some things and not others—but if this is true, do you need the social-learning story at all?

A better theory of the development of disgust takes as its starting point the observation of Darwin: disgust is at root a biological adaptation that evolved as a result of the benefits it gave our ancestors long ago.

This evolutionary theory leaves plenty of room for development. Not every ability that has evolved shows up early in a person's life. The physical ability to conceive children is an obvious example of this, along with the corresponding emotional and motivational systems that drive us to seek out and evaluate sexual partners. In the case of disgust, natural selection would not be so cruel as to curse babies to lie in misery, unable to move away from their own waste and perpetually disgusted as a result. And so it is not surprising that children in their first couple of years of life, in a situation where their mobility is limited and in which adults control their food intake, are free of disgust.

And young children really are disgust-free. Any parent will observe that they are entirely mellow about their own waste products. Rozin and his colleagues find that up until their third birthday, children will happily gobble up most anything they are offered—including grasshoppers and something they believe to be "dog doo" (it was actually a combination of peanut butter and cheese).

Once the innate disgust reaction kicks in, certain substances are universally found to be disgusting. The onset of disgust can happen quite suddenly. It is a lot like fear. There is a point in development at which previously fearless children often become intensely frightened of certain things—darkness, enclosed spaces, and spiders, for instance (which are the very same things that other primates are afraid of).

I first saw disgust emerge in Max when he was about three and a half years of age. I was changing my son Zachary's diaper on the living-room floor, and Max stood above me, watching with curiosity. The diaper was rather pungent, and Max looked unhappy and then started to gag. I asked him what was wrong, and he said, "My tummy hurts." I asked him why, and he said that he didn't know, and finally I gently moved him to another room. Surprisingly, Max was disgusted before he had any conscious insight into what he was disgusted by. Zachary began to show disgust at almost exactly the same age. He started to complain about certain bad smells, to wrinkle up his nose, and so on.

Disgust also requires learning. Unchanging facts about the world are plausible candidates for being hard-wired into the brain. This includes the foundational appreciation of objects and people, because wherever you are, it pays to think about the world in terms of objects that are solid and persist through time, and people who have goals and emotions. But other facts about the world change over the course of generations, too fast for biological evolution to keep up with. The personalities of the specific people you meet have to be learned, and so does the spatial environment in which you live. Similarly, if disgust is to serve its role of steering us away from bad meat, learning needs to be involved, since the sorts of foods that are toxic vary according to the local conditions. So although some things, such as feces, are universally repellent as foods because these are always bad for you to eat, there is going to be some variation as well, since the danger level of certain foods in a given environment cannot be specified by natural selection.

HOW TO DISGUST A CHILD

You might think, then, that the task for the evolutionary biologist, the developmental psychologist, and the cultural anthropologist is to find out what is universal, and then to answer the question: How do children learn what things are disgusting?

But this is not the right question. The class of things to learn about is the nondisgusting. Steven Pinker has observed, "Of all the parts of all the animals in creation, people eat an infinitesimal fraction, and everything else is untouchable. Many Americans eat only the skeletal muscle of cattle, chickens, swine, and a few fish. Other parts, like guts, brains, kidneys, eyes, and feet, are beyond the pale, and so is any part of any animal not on the list: dogs, pigeons, jellyfish, slugs, toads, insects, and the other millions of animal species." And Darwin also observed how cautious we are toward novel foods: "It is remarkable how readily and instantly retching or actual vomiting is induced in some persons by the mere idea of having partaken in any unusual food, as of an animal which is not commonly eaten, though there is nothing in such food to cause the stomach to reject it."

The question to ask, then, is: How does the child learn what is *not* disgusting?

Consider the following answer, in part based on research by the anthropologist Elizabeth Cashdan. Children start off without disgust. But by roughly their third birthday children get picky, and prefer to only eat foods that they have eaten previously. By their fourth birthday they are even pickier. By then, all meat that has not been previously experienced elicits disgust. And at this point, they have much the same intuitions about disgusting foods as adults do. They know that milk and potato chips make for fine foods, but when offered a grasshopper or "dog doo," they decline.

Since parents control young children's intake, this early period of openness to new foods allows them to shape their child's future preferences. This is what psychologists call a "sensitive period"—a span of time during which learning can most easily take place. Cashdan discovered that children who are introduced to solid foods unusually late tended to eat from a smaller selection of foods during childhood, presumably because the duration of this sensitive period was shortened; they had less time to try out new foods.

Are children's reactions here really disgust, in the same sense that the adults' reaction counts as disgust? The key test here has to do with contamination: if something is thought of as disgusting, then it should taint anything that it touches. To explore whether children understand this, the psychologist Michael Siegal and his colleagues did a series of studies with Australian three- and four-year-olds.

In one study, during snack time, the children were shown a drink with a cockroach floating on top of it. The adult said, "Here's some juice. Oh! It has a cockroach in it." And then the adult removed the cockroach, and asked, "Is the juice okay or not okay to drink?" Most of the children said it was not okay. They also said that other children would not want to drink the contaminated drink, and that other children would prefer to drink water than contaminated chocolate milk, even though chocolate milk is normally preferable.

In another study, children were tested on their moral reasoning in the realm of contamination. Jean Piaget and other developmental psychologists have maintained that young children do not appreciate the difference between a lie and a mistake—they are said to regard all false statements as lies. To explore this, an experiment was done in which children were shown moldy bread, and then the experimenter put Vegemite (an Australian breakfast spread) over the mold so as to hide it. There were two teddy bears present during this event, and children were told two scenarios and asked to differentiate between a lie and a mistake:

This bear didn't see the mold on the bread. He told a friend
       that it was okay to eat. Did the bear lie or make a mistake?
This bear did see the mold on the bread. He told a friend that
       it was okay to eat. Did the bear make a mistake or lie?

Young children tended to get this right: they understood that the first bear made a mistake and the second bear lied. And they later described the second bear, but not the first, as "naughty."

It is revealing that this fine-tuned moral sensitivity seems to exist only in the domain of contamination. In parallel situations, children didn't do as well. When, instead of moldy bread, there is a snake in a house and one bear sees the snake but says there is no snake, young children are nowhere near as good as figuring out this bear is a liar.

Expanding one's food preferences past the age of four is fraught with difficulty, even for adults. Research in this area has been done with military personnel, prompted by practical considerations: during World War II, American pilots in the Pacific went hungry because they refused to eat insects and toads, even though they had been explicitly taught that these foods were safe. Also, you can actually order military personnel, unlike college undergraduates, to do unpleasant things.

The consistent finding is that while you can force adults to eat novel foods—fried grasshoppers in one study—they are not happy about it. When adults do willingly try new foods, the foods are not really that different from old foods: if you like bread, and you like chocolate, you might cheerfully try chocolate bread. (In fact, up until the age of four, American children seem to have the rule that if they like A and they like B, they will like A+B, leading to interesting combinations such as whipped cream and hamburger or ice cream with ketchup on top.) We also sometimes try new foods if there is some other motivation at work, such as a desire to look tough, or to fit into a new group, or, of course, intense hunger. And of all the new foods to try, the hardest to stomach are those made of meat.

I had my own experience with this when I took my children to an edible insect show at a museum in New Haven. On stage, the "chef" fried up crickets in garlic and oil, placed them in little cups on top of some orzo pasta, and passed them around the audience. (He then said, repeatedly, "Bug Appetit!") Just about all children happily dug in. Some adults did too, but many refused, and one woman looked into her cup and *screamed*. I was confident that I would indulge, but when I saw the crickets, I froze, and had to put the cup down. Intellectually I had no problems, but I could not bring myself to act. Never underestimate the power of disgust.

THE SCOPE OF DISGUST

Disgust goes beyond the range of food, extending to death, violations of the "body envelope" (amputations, surgery, and so on), bad hygiene, and certain sex acts. Consider this list of scenarios, given to college undergraduates who were asked to rate them on how disgusting they are:

You see a bowel movement left unflushed in a public toilet.
Your friend's pet cat dies, and you have to pick up the dead
body with your bare hands.

You hear about an adult woman who has sex with her father.

You discover that a friend of yours changes underwear only
    once a week.

You see a man with his intestines exposed after an accident.

All of these items were judged as highly disgusting. Why? What property do they share?

The most elegant theory has been developed by Rozin, originally with April Fallon, and later with Jonathan Haidt and Robert McCauley. He suggests that disgust starts off as a rejection response to certain potential foods, and that it has evolved through natural selection for that purpose. But in the course of development it moves from a defense of the physical body to a more abstract defense of the soul. In particular, anything that reminds us that we are animals elicits disgust:

> Humans must eat, excrete, and have sex, just like animals. Each culture prescribes the proper way to perform these actions—by, for example, placing most animals off limits as potential foods and most people off limits as potential sexual partners. People who ignore these prescriptions are reviled as disgusting and animal-like. Furthermore, humans are like animals in having fragile body envelopes that, when breached, reveal blood and soft viscera; and human bodies, like animal bodies, die. Envelope violations and death are disgusting because they are uncomfortable reminders of our animal vulnerability. Finally, hygienic rules govern the proper use and maintenance of the human body, and the failure to meet these culturally defined standards places a person below the level of humans. Insofar as humans behave like animals, the distinction between human and animals is blurred, and we see ourselves as lowered, debased, and (perhaps most critically) mortal.

Because of this, Rozin describes disgust as "the body and soul emotion."

There are two deep insights here. The first is that the extension of disgust is a "preadaptation," something that has evolved for one purpose and is subsequently used for another purpose. The second is that we can be disgusted by people by virtue of our kinship to animals; we are not angels; we are meaty things.

But Rozin's theory is too conceptual, too cognitive. It misses the physicality, the sensuality, of disgust. It is just not such a smart emotion. Simply being reminded—intellectually—of the fact we are animals is neither necessary or sufficient for disgust. Humans breathe and sleep, after all, "just like animals." But breathing and sleeping are not disgusting. Looking at a brain scan or an X-ray is a stark and striking reminder of our physical nature, but these are not disgusting activities. Ruminating that I will one day die—just like any other animal—might make me sad, but it does not normally disgust me. In general, being reminded of our animal nature is not, by itself, disgusting.

A more plausible view is that death, bad hygiene, body-envelope violations, and certain sex acts disgust us simply because we perceive them, at a basic sensory level, in much the same way we perceive rotten meat and decaying flesh. This is most obvious in connection with death. Death itself is not disgusting. It is corpses that disgust us. Corpses are revolting not because their presence forces us to contemplate in some airy way our mortal nature. Corpses disgust us because they are rotting flesh. Violations of the bodily envelope disgust us not because they show us the fragility of our corporeal state, or because they indicate our kinship with other creatures. Such violations disgust us because they involve the very things that disgust has evolved to keep us away from: blood, pus, and soft tissue. Bad hygiene does not offend because we see the person as animal-like in his behavior. It offends because someone with bad hygiene smells bad, a smell disturbingly reminiscent of bad food. (There may be an additional consideration here, in that bad hygiene is a sign of disease.) Finally, sex typically involves contact with parts of the body associated with urine and feces, and so it is a particularly fecund area for disgust.

The argument so far is that disgust is limited to sensual domains—to a class of things that strike our senses in a certain way; it is not a thoughtful cognitive process. But the language of disgust does seem to apply to other sorts of things, far afield of the world of meat and waste:

> That idea really *stinks*.
> The way he weasels his way out of doing any work *makes me sick*.
> The high pay of CEOs is *revolting*.

In just a few months, I heard the word "disgusting" used to describe:

> The president's tax plan
> Someone writing a negative review of a grant proposal because
>   he disliked the applicant
> Microsoft
> The high cost of prepared spaghetti sauce

When people are asked to list what they find disgusting, they include not only the usual suspects (feces and the like), but also certain types of people, such as con men, Nazis, sexists, liberals, and conservatives. In a seminar on this topic, one graduate student insisted that a certain politician's statements during a televised debate nauseated her; had she continued to watch the debate, she was definitely "going to barf."

This all seems to indicate that disgust can be highly abstract and intellectual. But I am skeptical. My hunch is that in these statements "disgust" is a metaphor. Saying that we are disgusted by a tax plan is like saying that we are thirsty for knowledge or lusting after a new car. After all, if you actually observe people's faces and actions during heated political or academic discourse, you will witness a lot of anger, even hate, but rarely, if ever, the facial or emotive signs of disgust.

To say that this is a metaphor is not to dismiss it as unimportant. It is a pervasive metaphor, and one of considerable power. As Miller notes, "No other emotion, not even hatred, paints its object so unflatteringly." Suppose I wish to attack a certain theory of child development. It is one thing to describe it as stupid or incoherent or to go on about how angry it makes me. But to describe it as disgusting ups the ante. It renders the thing that I am talking about objectively and concretely vile, and it taints whoever endorses it.

When you say that such-and-so is disgusting, you give the impression that this would be apparent to any normal observer. It is like saying that it is bigger than a breadbox. To say that something is disgusting is to imply, "If you were to see it, you would find it disgusting too." (If you don't, there is something wrong *with you*.) There is no response to the language of disgust. It is a conversation stopper.

An example of how disgust can be used to attack certain views is from the ethicist Leon Kass's recent discussion of human cloning. After conceding that "revulsion is not an argument," he goes on to say:

> In some crucial cases, however, repugnance is the emotional expression of deep wisdom, beyond wisdom's power completely to articulate it. Can anyone really give an argument fully adequate to the horror that is father-daughter incest (even with consent), or bestiality, or the mutilation of a corpse, or the rape or murder of another human being? Would anybody's failure to give full rational justification for his revulsion at these practices make that revulsion ethically suspect?
>
> I suggest that our repugnance at human cloning belongs in this category. We are repelled by the prospect of cloning human beings not because of the strangeness or the novelty of the undertaking, but

because we intuit and we feel, immediately and without argument, the violation of things that we rightfully hold dear.

Miller himself makes a similar argument, in his contribution to a series of essays sparked by the successful cloning of Dolly, a sheep.

> I am, it should by now be clear, disgusted, even revolted by the idea of cloning: not just the idea of cloning humans, but the idea of cloning sheep too. I am quite frankly disgusted by Dolly. . . . All I mean to say is that there are certain large constraints on being human and we have certain emotions that tell us when we are pressing against these constraints in a dangerous way. This is part of the job that disgust, horror, and the sense of the uncanny do; they tell us when we are leaving the human for something else; either downward toward the material, mechanical, and bestial; or upward toward the realm of spirit or the world of pure hokum.

But it is just not true that we react to cloning in the same way that we do to incest, corpse mutilation, and bestiality. Many people think human cloning is a bad idea, even a terrible idea, but this is not the same as feeling revulsion. Perhaps you took the kids to see Arnold Schwarzenegger in the popular movie *The Sixth Day*? (Arnold goes to clone the family pet, and then, through sinister machinations, *he* gets cloned!) I would be surprised if Columbia Pictures were to release a popular action film around the theme of bestiality. Indeed, when Peter Singer in an article called "Heavy Petting" dared to discuss the moral issues surrounding bestiality (in order to make a point about the inconsistency in how we treat animals), the response was ridicule and anger. Certain topics are taboo. Cloning is not one of them.

I do not doubt that Kass, Miller, and many others are convinced that cloning is wrong, and that their conviction might be the result of an intuition that they might not be able fully to articulate. But unless they are unusual, their responses to cloning are not revulsion, repugnance, or disgust as we normally experience them.

I suspect that Kass is well aware of this. He is not reminding us of our disgust; he is trying to *elicit* it, through phrases such as "a radical form of child abuse," "our horror at human cloning," and so on. He is trying to persuade people that they *should* respond to cloning in this way, and that it is a moral failing if they do not. If most people think of cloning as akin to bestiality, then what sort of monster are you to favor it? As he intones ominously, "Shallow are the souls that have forgotten how to shudder."

Even if Kass were right, and we really did find human cloning revolting, it is not clear what would follow from this. Contrary to what Kass and Miller imply, revulsion is not always the expression of deep wisdom, nor is it a useful tool for detecting when we are violating constraints on being human. It can be a cruel and stupid emotion. Through American history, many have found the notion of interracial sex to be disgusting, a reaction that has found its expression in lynching. And revulsion has often found targets in groups of people—women, homosexuals, Jews, untouchables, and so on. Of the emotions that one could use as a moral guide, I would prefer sympathy, compassion, and pity.

DISGUSTING PEOPLE

Would you wear someone else's clothes? What if the person has experienced an amputation, or suffered from a disease like tuberculosis? What about a moral taint—would you wear Hitler's sweater? Timothy McVeigh's baseball cap? Many people say no. In fact, even if the item is fully cleaned and comes from a normal, healthy, morally acceptable person, many of us still prefer not to wear a stranger's clothes. We are easily disgusted by other people. This propensity has troubling, sometimes horrific, social consequences.

The philosopher Martha Nussbaum offers the following summary of how disgust has been used as a weapon:

> Thus, throughout history, certain disgust properties—sliminess, bad smell, stickiness, decay, foulness—have repeatedly and monotonously been associated with, indeed projected onto, groups by reference to whom privileged groups seek to define their superior human status. Jews, women, homosexuals, untouchables, lower-class people—all of these are imagined as tainted by the dirt of the body.

The Jews have long been a target of disgust. First Jews themselves have been said to be disgusting. Voltaire wrote, "The Jews were more subject to leprosy than any other people living in hot climates, because they had neither linen, nor domestic baths. These people were so negligent of cleanliness and the decencies of life that their legislators were obliged to make a law to compel them even to wash their hands." It was claimed that Jewish males menstruated. Second, Jews did disgusting things to cherished people and objects. They used the blood of Christian children in rituals. In 1215, the doctrine of transmutation was established as dogma, and in prompt response to this, Jews were said to have desecrated the Host, spitting and defecating on it.

The perception of certain groups as disgusting leads directly to the topic of genocide. There are many causes of genocide, including the belief that members of the targeted group are enemies of God, or an ongoing threat, or that they have committed some atrocity in the past, one that demands vengeance. But disgust has a special status. It is a remarkable fact of human psychology that disgust is a very effective way to motivate people towards mass murder, and appears to have been used in every genocide in recorded history.

This might seem puzzling. It makes sense to tell people that their targets are dangerous, or that their targets did terrible things to them in the past. But why tell them that these people are disgusting?

The simplest answer is that disgust is a negative emotion, one associated with repugnant things, and by stating that certain people are disgusting, you inspire negative thoughts toward them. But a better answer goes right to the heart of intuitive dualism. Disgust is a response to people's bodies, not to their souls. If you see people as souls, they have moral worth: You can hate them and hold them responsible; you can view them as evil; you can love them and forgive them, and see them as blessed. They fall within the moral circle. But if you see them solely as bodies, they lose any moral weight. Empathy does not extend to them. And so dictators and warmongers have come across the insight, over and over again, that you can get people to commit the most terrible atrocities using the tool of disgust.

The clearest modern example of how this works comes from Nazi propaganda, which described the Jews as dirty, filthy, disease-ridden; they were portrayed as rats, garbage, and bacillus, agents of infection. As Nussbaum put it, "The stock image of the Jew, in anti-Semitic propaganda, was that of a being disgustingly soft and porous, receptive of fluid and sticky, womanlike in its oozy sliminess, a foul parasite inside the clean body of the German male self." The Turks said similar things about the Armenians in the 1920s, as did the Hutus about the Tutsis in Rwanda in the 1990s.

One strategy of oppressors during acts of genocide is to arrange the world so as to make their victims act and appear disgusting. In the course of starving Armenian families nearly to death, their tormentors would speak with disdain about the "clawlike hands" of the Armenians, fighting for food like "ravenous dogs." And the Nazis, having trapped the Jews in conditions in which hygiene was difficult or impossible—as in the concentration camps and, to a lesser extent, the ghettos—would speak with satisfaction of their filthiness. Primo Levi describes Jews' being denied access to toilets, and the reaction that this prompted:

The SS escort did not hide their amusement at the sight of men and women squatting wherever they could, on the platforms and in the middle of the tracks, and the German passengers openly expressed their disgust: people like this deserve their fate, look at how they behave. These are not *Menschen,* human beings, but animals, it's as clear as day.

Terrence Des Pres has argued that many of those who survived the concentration camps were people who took great care to keep themselves as clean as possible, so as to retain their dignity, both to themselves and to others, in the face of attempts to make them appear like beasts.

Disgust is not the only way to diminish people. One can also try to rob them of individuality—describing them as "cargo," designating them by number, and so on. (Hence the wisdom of the framers of the Convention on the Rights of the Child to state that every child has the right to a proper name.) Humor can also be used to dehumanize by making people laughable. During the Cultural Revolution, people were paraded through the street with dunce caps, or made to wear placards with degrading slogans on them. But disgust is the tool usually used to dehumanize; it is visceral and potent.

Disgust can be used as well for more exalted purposes. Some have tried to motivate a spiritual existence, or a life of the soul, by eliciting a negative reaction to our material bodies. St. Augustine was greatly influenced by Cicero's vivid image of Etruscan pirates' torture of prisoners by strapping a corpse to them face to face. This, Augustine maintained, is the fate of the soul, chained to a physical body as one would be chained to a rotting corpse.

What are the limits to disgust?

Consider sex. Just as with food, it would be a mistake to ask which sex acts are disgusting. There are just too many. There is sex with animals, sex with children and babies, sex with dead bodies.

Some are revolted by homosexual sex, by sex of the old or even middle-aged, by sex between people of different races, by sex involving people with disabilities; some would be appalled to observe masturbation, or certain sexual activities or even certain positions. Even cheerful and conventional heterosexual sex between consenting adults, even very attractive consenting adults, can easily be seen as disgusting at least some of the time. To try to list all the disgusting sexual acts perversion by perversion, position by position, and ascertain what property they share is the wrong research project.

On a parallel with food, the right question is: Which sex acts are *not* disgusting? The humorist Stephen Fry provides one answer. After outlining what he sees as the bestial nature of sexual intimacy—"I would be greatly in the debt of the man who could tell me what would ever be appealing about those damp, dark, foulsmelling and revoltingly tufted areas of the body that constitute the main dishes in the banquet of love"—he notes that sexual arousal overrides any more civilized reticence: "Once under the influence of the drugs supplied by one's own body, there is no limit to the indignities, indecencies, and bestialities to which the most usually rational and graceful of us will sink." In other words, lust can trump disgust.

At this point, we can clear up something that puzzled Freud, that "a man who will kiss a pretty girl's mouth passionately, may perhaps be disgusted by the idea of using her tooth-brush." Freud used this as an example of how irrational the emotion of disgust is, but it is easily explained: In the act of kissing, sexual arousal plays a role, and this blocks disgust. There is a parallel here with hunger; people who are starving will eat most anything, including human flesh.

Lust has its own moral problems. It is hardly a new insight that there can be a tension between viewing someone with sexual desire and viewing them as a person with moral worth. Feminists have long written about the immorality of seeing someone "as an object," and I think the phrase here is particularly apt. Obviously, lust and love can coexist, but it is disturbing how easily lust, like disgust, can block an appreciation of a person as a person. The worry here was summed up, with some bitterness, by Marilyn Monroe, who once said, "I have never liked sex. I do not think I ever will. It seems just the opposite of love."

What about love, then? Love defeats disgust as well, but in a very different way. When you love a person, you see the person not as a body but as a soul. In his studies of why some marriages last and others break up, the psychologist John Gottman found the major signal that a marriage was in trouble. It is not heated argument or stony silence. It is when disgust, and its kin, contempt, shows itself.

Christian theology is chock full of saints and revered people who express their love of humanity and God by doing things that others find repulsive, such as washing the bodies of filthy strangers, caring for lepers, and, in the case of St. Catherine, engaging in acts that I cannot bear to describe. But there are more mundane examples of relatively repugnant acts that we do out of love. Changing the diaper of a child is a common one, as is caring for an elderly relative. Disgust is not absent in such cases, but it is diminished. I found it much easier to change the diaper of my own child than of another's, and much of this, I think, is because of love. In his discussion of how doctors operate on patients, the surgeon Atul Gawande describes an attitude of "tenderness and aestheticism" toward the body as both a person deserving of respect and a problem to be solved. (Note, incidentally, that disgust is just one emotion that needs to be tempered during medical procedures; sexual desire is another.)

There are other, more mundane psychological processes whereby disgust is set aside. There is habituation—the dullness of a response upon repeated exposures. You get used to certain things, and they come to bother you less. And people also exercise some control over how they encounter the potentially disgusting. When changing a diaper, they are careful to avert their eyes, breathe through the mouth, and think of other things. On a more cognitive level, one really can go mad worrying about rat droppings on one's food, the true composition of hot dogs, and so on, and we just try to not dwell on such matters. This is not always successful: On a trip to London, I had the bad luck to read a newspaper report describing how scientists analyzed bowls of beer nuts from British pubs and discovered that they are inevitably covered with a thin coating of urine, due to drinkers who are less than fastidious about washing their hands after using the toilet. I was unable to avoid dwelling on this while in pubs, and often stared unhappily as others gobbled down these snacks.

Finally, there are social structures in place that have emerged in order to shield the disgusting from us, to hide it from our eyes, or to reassure us about borderline cases. This is a function of manners. One example comes from a book of conduct written in 1558, which states: "You should not offer your handkerchief to anyone unless it has been freshly washed. . . nor is it seemly, to spread out your handkerchief and peer into it as if pearls and rubies might have fallen out of your head." It is a function of certain religion laws, such as the rule that if a kosher food is somehow contaminated, the food remains acceptable so long as the contaminant is less than one sixtieth the volume of the total. And it is a function of euphemism. Americans and Europeans go to great pains to hide the origins of our foods both by the way we prepare them and by the way we speak of them, using terms like "beef" and "pork." (A friend of mine tells the story of her daughter, who once observed with some fascination, "Isn't it interesting that we call this food 'lamb'? That's the same name as real lambs!" She was horrified to hear that this is not coincidental, and is still—more than a decade later—a vegetarian.)

Other social structures exist to present us with the disgusting in carefully controlled doses. Universally disgusting things often show up in rituals. The Nuer bathe in cow urine, the Zunis have a ritual in which they eat dog feces, and members of the Skull and Bones club at Yale are rumored to have an initiation rite that involves lying naked in a coffin, buried in mud. Doing something that is unpleasant serves as a test of one's loyalty, and it establishes group solidarity through shared suffering. Contact with disgusting substances serves as an excellent mechanism through which to establish such suffering.

Overall, disgust does exert a bit of a fascination. Jonathan Haidt points out that when you ask someone, "Do you want to see something disgusting?" the answer is almost always a cautious "Yes." All negative emotions have this appeal. We poke at sores, go on amusement park rides that terrify us, see tragedies that make us cry. Freudians might see some pathology in all this, but I am more inclined to credit Rozin's "benign masochism" theory, which is that we train ourselves to encounter the world—to see what we can do and what our limits are—by sometimes confronting ourselves with negative experiences that are under our control and that pose no real threat.

Finally, disgust is a great source of humor. Some commentators see gross-out humor as a recent invention, but classic Greek comedies were filled with this sort of thing; there was no shortage of bathroom humor in Aristophanes. Any good theory of comedy has to explain why.

THE UNBEARABLE LIGHTNESS OF BEAN

Before we ask the question of what disgust and humor have in common, let's pursue a broader question: What makes us laugh? A popular book on the brain makes this confident claim: "We laugh when there is incongruity between what we expect and what actually happens, unless the outcome is frightening." But this cannot be right. Incongruity is clearly an aspect of humor, but it is not enough. Finding a shoe in a dishwasher is incongruous, and so is snow in

July, but they are not in and of themselves funny. The incongruity has to be of a certain type.

Arthur Koestler narrowed down the incongruity theory by pointing out that the essence of humor involves a shift in perspective—the punch line is incongruous within the original frame of reasoning but makes sense within a different frame, as in these examples:

When is a door not a door?
  When it is a jar!

Do you know beer makes you smarter?
  It made Budweiser!

The humor here comes from shifts in perspective. Suppose the response to the first question were "When it is a chicken!" This is incongruous, but not funny, because it makes no sense at all. But the double meaning in the punch line "a jar" makes it a joke.

We are getting closer, but there is a problem with this theory of humor. These jokes are not funny. They elicit groans. If they make someone laugh, they most likely do so just because they are so bad. This sort of verbal humor—along with knock-knock jokes, light bulb jokes, and elephant jokes—is at best clever. They are joke wannabes, meeting the formal criteria but lacking the certain ingredient that makes a joke truly funny.

The missing ingredient is a certain type of wickedness. No serious student of laughter could miss its cruel nature. The psychologist Robert Provine notes that despite laughter's sometimes gentle reputation, it can be an outrageously vicious sound. Not so long ago, the elite would find it endlessly amusing to visit insane asylums and laugh at the inmates; physical and mental deformity has always been a source of amusement. There was no shortage of laughter at public executions and floggings, and the sound is often an accompaniment to raping, looting, and killing in time of war. During the massacre of high school students at Littleton, Colorado, the killers laughed. I once saw a terrible picture of a small Jewish boy in the Germany of World War II, on his knees, forced to scrub the street; the adults around him were laughing and jeering. Many reports of torture involve humiliating the victim in ways that are comical to his or her tormentors. A veteran of World War II reported how his unit found a hiding Japanese soldier and used him for target practice, firing at him as he ran frantically around a clearing: "They found his movements hilarious and their laughter slowed down their eventual killing of him. They were cheered by the incident and joked about it for days." This same aggression shows up even in primate equivalents of this human act. Gangs of monkeys make laughter-like sounds when they attack a common enemy. And chimpanzees, like humans, make laughing sounds when acting in mock aggression.

We're getting there, but it is too simple to see humor as a shifting frame of reference with an added dash of cruelty. It needs to be the right type of cruelty. The comic Mel Brooks once said, "Tragedy is when I cut my finger. Comedy is when you fall into an open sewer and die." And Dave Barry puts it best in this advice to aspiring humor writers:

> "The most important humor truth of all is that to really see the humor in a situation, you have to have perspective. 'Perspective' is derived from two ancient Greek words: 'persp' meaning 'something bad that happens to somebody else' and 'ective' meaning 'ideally someone like Donald Trump.'"

The important ingredient here is a loss of dignity; someone is knocked off his pedestal, brought down a peg. Laughter can serve as a weapon, one that can be used by a mob. It is contagious and involuntary; it has great subversive power, so much so that Plato thought it should be banned from the state. But also, in gentler hands, it can signal playfulness and establish friendship. You can puncture your own dignity, and can laugh—and make others laugh—at yourself.

Humor can also have a particularly direct relationship to the interplay between bodies and souls. Humor involves a shift in perspective, and one of the most striking shifts is when we move from seeing someone as a sentient being, a soul, to seeing the person as merely a body. Henri Bergson proposed that humor is based on this body/soul duality—what he called "something mechanical encrusted upon the living" and what Koestler called "the dualism of subtle mind and inert matter." Plainly a lot of humor has nothing to do with bodies and souls, but there is one domain in which this dualism reigns supreme. This is slapstick.

In his study of American slapstick, Alan Dale notes that every funny act falls into one of two categories—the blow and the fall. The canonical blow is a pie in the face and the canonical fall is caused by a banana peel, but the categories are quite broad, corresponding to either an intentional assault upon the hero's dignity (blow) or its involuntary collapse (fall). In *Dumb and Dumber,* Jeff Daniels succumbs to a violent attack of diarrhea owing to the comically abundant dose of laxatives that Jim Carrey has slipped into his food. This is a blow. In *Bean,* Rowan Atkinson is admiring a priceless work of art, smiling and humming cheerfully to himself, when he suddenly and explosively sneezes all over it. This is a fall.

Disgust, religion, and slapstick all traffic in what Dale calls "the debasing effect of the body on the soul." But they do so in different ways. Disgust focuses on the body, dismissing the soul; religion, at least some of the time, focuses on the soul and rejects the body. And slapstick is the richest of all, as it deals with both at the same time, showing a person with feeling and goals trapped in a treacherous physical shell. As Dale puts it, slapstick has a "secular sense of the soul encased in the body that only holds it back."

This might seem like a fancy analysis of why we laugh when someone gets hit by a pie or slips on a banana peel. But without this duality, slapstick fails—there is no humor at all. It is revealing, then, that young children immediately appreciate this sort of humor. If you are in a bind and need to make a two-year-old laugh, the best way to do so is to adopt a surprised expression and fall on your ass.

PART IV

THE SPIRITUAL REALM

7

THEREFORE I AM

"Pig valves." Rabbit tries to hide his revulsion. "Was it
terrible? They split your chest open and run your blood
through a machine?"

"Piece of cake. You're knocked out cold. What's
wrong with running your blood through a machine?
What else you think you are, champ?"

A god-made one-of-a-kind with an immortal soul
breathed in. A vehicle of grace. A battlefield of good
and evil. An apprentice angel.

—John Updike, *Rabbit at Rest*

Always go to other people's funerals, otherwise they
won't come to yours.

—Yogi Berra

WHEN SOMEONE DIES, how do you keep the soul from reanimat-
ing the body? After all, the person is not going to be pleased to leave
the world of friends, family, and possessions, and will naturally struggle to get his or her body back. As the archaeologist Timothy Taylor
points out, this is the same impulse that would lead you to pick up a

valuable object that was knocked from your hands. But the reanimation of the body is bad news for those who remain, since the damaged
and decaying corpse might try to take back its possessions, including
its spouse. Many societies have developed ingenious methods so as to
enchant the soul, frighten it off, or distract it from its mission.

This is only a temporary problem. As the body decomposes, the
soul moves further toward the spirit world, and once enough time
has passed (such as when the flesh is entirely gone from the bones),
reanimation becomes increasingly unlikely—though there is often
the need for secondary rites, sometimes weeks or months later, to
make sure that the soul remains firmly in the realm of the ancestors.
This is one reason for the "double funerals" that are common in
many cultures; there is one set of rituals immediately after death,
and then a second set so as to hasten the soul to a final resting place.

Most readers of this book have never worried about how to keep
a soul from repossessing a corpse. Reanimation is the stuff of horror
movies. But the worry is not entirely alien; it is an unusual variation
on a common theme. More familiar versions include the notion
that the soul might ascend to heaven, plummet to hell, or occupy
the body of another animal or person. If you do not believe that you
can communicate with the dead, or that you should pray for the
soul's safekeeping, then I imagine you know someone who does.

When directly asked, most Americans say that they believe in
Heaven (90 percent), hell (73 percent) and angels (72 percent).
Most state that they look forward to meeting their friends and family members in heaven, and about one in six go further and claim
that they already have been in contact with someone who has died.

To my knowledge, nobody has systematically asked people about
the more general premise of a body/soul duality, about whether they
agree with John Updike's character Rabbit. Do you believe that you
are (A) a machine or (B) an immaterial soul? (B) is the aesthetically
appealing choice. (Who would prefer the claim of Marvin Minsky, a

pioneer in the field of artificial intelligence, that we are nothing more than "meat machines"?) We do not feel as if we *are* bodies; we feel as if we *occupy* them. Some might wish to answer "all of the above," self-identifying as both a body and as a soul. But only a small minority would choose just (A).

What can be said about this minority view, one subscribed to by many psychologists and neuroscientists? I do not doubt the sincerity of such an answer. But I would put those who reject dualism in the same category as those who, through scientific reasoning or philosophical deliberations, come to believe that there is no external world, just sensory impressions (as did Bishop Berkeley), or that thoughts and feelings do not exist (as some radical behaviorists assert), or that there is no such thing as morality, or truth, or pain. These scientists and philosophers might be perfectly sincere in these beliefs. But such views are held at an airy intellectual level, slapped on top of our foundational appreciation that the world contains objects, minds, morals, truth, and experience. At this gut level, souls exist.

The premise of this book is that we are dualists who have two ways of looking at the world: in terms of bodies and in terms of souls. A direct consequence of this dualism is the idea that bodies and souls are separate. And from this follow certain notions that we hold dear, including the concepts of self, identity, and life after death.

WHAT YOU KNOW FOR SURE

Try for a minute to be a philosophical skeptic. Normal skeptics doubt the existence of ESP, poltergeists, UFOs and the life-enhancing powers of green tea, but you put these skeptics to shame. You doubt just about everything. For instance, most people accept that they have lived for years. But you might wonder whether the universe had been created seconds ago, and all your memories are illusions. In science fiction, robots and full-grown clones are created believing they have had parents, a childhood, a rich life—but they are mistaken; their memories are false. (Think *Blade Runner.*) How can you be sure that this is not true of you?

You can certainly doubt that you have a brain. Young children toddle on quite happily without knowing that they have one, and most humans have lived and died without ever knowing that such an organ existed. Even once the brain was discovered, it was a while before anyone knew what it was for—the ancient Greeks thought its main function was to cool the blood.

Although now even the most devout would agree that the brain is intimately related to mental and spiritual life—the seat of the soul, perhaps—this was not always so clear. In the fifteenth century, the Church struggled with the question of whether to baptize two-headed conjoined twins once or twice. Modern sensibilities say twice. The fact that there are two heads should make it plain that you are dealing with two people. But many felt that the soul resided in the heart, and the solution to the problem rested on the question of how many hearts there were. Ambroise Pare told of a baby brought to him after its death in 1546 that had two heads, two arms, and four legs. After dissecting the body Pare concluded, "I found but one heart by which one may know it was but one infant."

Contemporary scientists see the brain as the organ of thought. But as a skeptic you might take to heart (so to speak) a *Science* article written by Roger Lewin in 1980, "Is Your Brain Really Necessary?" in which he reported a case study of a student who was referred to the neuroscientist John Lorber because he had an unusually large head. Lorber reported that the student was highly intelligent and socially adept, but was unusual in one interesting regard: he had "virtually no brain. . . . When we did a brain scan on him. . . we saw that instead of the normal 4.5 centimeter thickness of brain tissue between the ventricles and the cortical surface, there was just a thin layer of mantle measuring a millimeter or so. His cranium is filled mainly with cerebrospinal fluid."

Of course he did have *some* brain, but the point of the article is that we might need less brain that we once thought. Lorber's report is controversial, and it is possible that the brain scan was done improperly. But it is certainly conceivable that Lorber was right. To the skeptic this would suggest that one day he might find an intelligent and social person with no brain at all!

You can doubt the existence of your entire body. There are cases of phantom limbs, in which someone feels pain in an amputated limb, and there are even cases in which there is the delusion that the limb really does still exist. How do you know that you do not have a phantom body? Or perhaps you are just a brain in a vat, and your so-called experiences are the results of electrical pulses engineered by a team of curious neuroscientists or sinister computers (think *The Matrix*). This is a modern version of a very old worry: hundreds of years ago, some of your skeptical counterparts worried that their experiences were induced by evil spirits.

In 1641, René Descartes set himself the project of philosophical skepticism, and subjected himself to the mental discipline of doubting everything he knew—from science, from experience, and even from the perception of his own body.

He observed that certain lunatics, "befogged by the black vapors of the bile," believe that they are kings, or that their heads are made out of clay, or that their bodies are glass. Although Descartes refused to entertain the possibility that he himself might be a lunatic, he noted that when he slept, he dreamed the same things that lunatics imagine while they are awake. So how could he be certain that he was not now asleep?

But there is one thing that Descartes could not doubt:

I have just convinced myself that nothing whatsoever existed in the world, that there was no sky, no earth, no minds, and no bodies;

have I not thereby convinced myself that I did not exist? Not at all. . . . Even though there may be a deceiver of some sort, very powerful and very tricky, who bends all his efforts to keep me perpetually deceived, there can be no slightest doubt that I exist, since he deceives me; and let him deceive me as much as he will, he can never make me nothing as long as I think I am something.

The one thing that is intuitively clear to us is our own existence as thinking beings. Descartes' pithy formulation of this conclusion is the most famous sentence in philosophy: *Cogito ergo sum.* I think, therefore I am.

Descartes asks, "What am I?" and he answers that though he cannot be sure that he is rational, or that he has a body, he knows he is a "thinking being. What is a thinking being? It is a being which doubts, which understands, which conceives, which affirms, which denies, which wills, which rejects, which imagines also, and which perceives."

Taking the next step, he concludes that since you can doubt the body but cannot doubt the self—"the soul"—the body is not necessary for the soul to exist. Furthermore, it is clear that the mind and body have different properties. The body is extended in space; the mind is not. The body is divisible; the mind is not. There are two distinct "substances": a body, which Descartes was perfectly content to think of as a "well-made clock," and a soul, which is immaterial and intangible.

Many philosophers have pointed out that this is not actually a good argument for a real duality of body and soul. The fact that we can imagine two things as being separate does not mean that they actually are separable. Imagination can be a poor guide to reality. It may also have been clear to Descartes that water is continuous at every level, and not made of particles, and perhaps he could also imagine a vehicle flying faster than light, or a loud noise in a vacuum. It would be a poor physics that took these intuitions as proof that such states of affairs are possible. Similarly, it would be a poor psychology that took the intuition that the body is not necessary for thought or that the mind is unextended and indivisible as proof that the body is, in fact, not necessary for thought and that the mind is, in fact, unextended and indivisible.

But the outcome of Descartes' exercise is a highly illuminating finding about common sense. He explores our basic intuitions about the proper answer to the question "Who am I?" And his answer is "I am not a body. I am a feeling, acting being that occupies a body."

This is how we see ourselves and others. Our bodies are described as our possessions. We talk about "my body," "my arm," "my heart," and, most revealingly, "my brain." The comedian Emo Phillips nicely captures the intuitive dichotomy between self and brain when he says, "I used to think the brain was the most fascinating part of the human body, but then I thought: 'Look what's telling me that!'"

Our intuitive dualism grounds our understanding of personal identity. We recognize that a person's body will age; it might grow or shrink, lose a limb, undergo plastic surgery—but in an important sense, the person remains the same. We will punish an old man for crimes he committed as a young man and will reward an 18-year-old with a fortune that was left to her as a baby. And we can understand fictional worlds in which a prince turns into a frog and then back into a prince again, or a vampire transforms to a bat. We can understand the passage in *The Odyssey* where the companions of Odysseus are magically transformed so that they "had the head, and voice, and bristles, and body of swine; but their mind remained unchanged as before. So they were penned there, weeping." We can make sense of Kafka's famous story that opens with the sentence, "As Gregor Samsa awoke one morning from uneasy dreams he found himself transformed in his bed into a gigantic insect."

Some people believe that more than one person can occupy a single body. In *The Exorcist* and other books and films of that genre, Satan struggles with the body's rightful owner. Most of us consider such stories fiction, but it is based on some people's sincere religious belief, and exorcisms are still being done. The secular equivalent of demonic possession is multiple-personality disorder (technically known as "dissociative identity disorder"), in which one body seems to be occupied by many "people" with different personalities, ages, and sexual proclivities.

Some artificial creatures are seen as possessing souls, often as a consequence of some transforming force, such as the bolt of lightning that animated Frankenstein's monster. Modern versions of such creations are robots and computers, some of whom, like the character Number 5 in the movie *Short Circuit,* are friendly childlike creatures, whereas others, like Proteus in the movie *Demon Seed,* are sinister entities that want to impregnate women. These are to be distinguished from soulless creatures such as Haitian zombies and the Jewish golem. According to Jewish tradition, the golem was a lump of clay that was animated to serve as a guardian for the Jews of medieval Prague. In Hebrew, *golem* means "shapeless mass" and, according to the Talmud, refers to bodies without souls. Zombies and golems are shambling robots that engage in complex behavior only when instructed to do so by another force.

Debates about animal rights and the potential of computers and robots are often approached by asking: Does a chimpanzee have a soul? Can a computer ever have a soul? There is even debate over whether clones have souls. In 1977, the Pontifical Academy of Life, established by Pope John Paul II, stated that souls can only be produced through God, raising the possibility that clones, created by man, would not have souls. The suggestion that clones are nothing special—merely identical twins born at different times—is apparently not convincing to everyone; some see the soul as an extra ingredient that must be added, and they worry that God might not bother.

The soul also has a part to play in the discussion of abortion. In a 1992 town meeting, President Clinton suggested that the abortion debate turns on when one thinks the soul enters the body. The position of the Roman Catholic church is that this occurs at the moment of conception, but other theologians have suggested that it enters at the moment of first movement—the "quickening"—or even days or weeks after birth.

If the universe contains souls as distinct entities *and* if some things have souls and others do not *and* if possession of a soul is necessary and sufficient to guarantee an entity's right to survive, there would be a simple way of thinking about certain significant moral problems. Debates over cloning, animal rights, and abortion would largely be reduced to determining whether the entity in question (clone, animal, fetus) has a soul. One of the many advantages of thinking about the world in terms of bodies and souls is the moral clarity that this provides.

Unfortunately this clarity is not justified. There is a sense in which souls exist, but they are not independent of bodies and brains. The qualities that we are most interested in from a moral standpoint—such as consciousness, experience of pain, and desire to thrive—are the result of brain processes, and such processes emerge gradually in both development and evolution. It is therefore unreasonable to seek an instant where they appear in development, or a sudden jump in the course of evolution.

An ironic consequence of a scientific perspective on mental life is that it takes the interesting moral questions away from the scientists. Researchers will be able to tell us with increasing precision about the mental and physical capacities of a zygote, fetus, embryo, and baby, as well as about the capacities of other species, information that is relevant when it comes to making certain moral decisions. But it does not itself settle the issues. Science does not answer the hard question of what capacities an entity must have to be included in the moral circle; to the extent that there is a line to be drawn, science does not tell us where to draw it.

As Steven Pinker points out, the discovery of the material basis of the soul changes the moral question. Our task is not to "discover" the moment in which someone becomes a person; it is to determine which qualities are deemed sufficiently important for us to extend certain rights and privileges. It is possible for two people to agree totally about the mental and physical capacities of an embryo, and yet for one to see abortion as acceptable and the other to see it as immoral. This is because they might have different views as to how much these capacities should be valued, and how they should be weighed against other considerations, such as the rights of the mother.

Does this mean that anything goes, there is no morality? Consider a parallel case. We have age restrictions as to when one is permitted to have sex, marry, serve in the military, or purchase alcohol. Presumably everyone would agree both that the optimal ages here are not to be solely determined by scientists, and that the boundaries are inherently fuzzy. There is no precise moment that separates those who are ready to fornicate or buy beer from those who are not. Does this mean that it would make perfect sense to raise the drinking age to 70, or lower the marriage age to 5? Of course not. Similarly, the lack of an objectively sharp boundary for moral values does not mean that distinctions do not exist. They do not force us to doubt that, say, five-year-olds really are people, deserving of life and respect, and clumps of dirt are not.

THE CARTESIAN CHILD

Jean Piaget believed that an understanding of the mental world is a late accomplishment, asserting, "The child cannot distinguish a real house, for example, from the concept or mental image or name of the house." But we know this to be mistaken. The psychologist Henry Wellman sums up the modern developmental evidence by saying, "My own position is that young children are dualists: knowledgeable of mental states and entities as ontologically different from physical objects and real events."

Wellman is not saying that young children know that they are dualists. Preschool children do not spontaneously mull over the mind/body problem. Even adults can live a full life without developing an explicit theory about the nature of experience and how it relates to the material world. Children are dualists in the same way that they are essentialists, realists, and moralists. They are dualists in the sense that they naturally see the world as containing two distinct domains, what Wellman calls "physical objects and real events" and "mental states and entities"—what I have described as bodies and souls.

Wellman's conclusion is based on a series of influential experiments. In one of them, young children were told stories involving mental entities versus physical entities. For instance, one tale was about one boy who had a cookie and another boy who was thinking about a cookie. Even three-year-olds understand the difference between a real cookie, which can be seen and touched by another person, and an imagined cookie, which cannot be; conversely, an imagined cookie can be mentally transformed by the person who is thinking about it, but a real cookie cannot be.

What do children know about where these mental states and entities come from? In our society children are explicitly taught about the brain and its role in thinking, but this understanding does not come easily. Piaget found that up until the age of about eight, the children he studied had little understanding of what the brain was for. Modern American and European children are more precocious than this. Five-year-olds know where the brain is and what it is for, and they know that people and other animals cannot think without a brain. But they do not usually understand that the brain is needed for physical action, such as hopping or brushing your teeth, and they do not think the brain is needed for an activity like pretending to be a kangaroo. And if you tell these children a story in which a child's brain is successfully transplanted into the head of a pig, children agree that the pig would now be as smart as a person, but they think that it would still keep the memories, personality, and identity of the pig.

I only really believed these findings when my six-year-old son, Max, expressed the same sentiments in the course of an argument. I was telling him that he had to go to bed, and he shouted at me that I could make him stay in his bed, but "you can't make me go to sleep—it's *my brain!*" I then sat down with him and asked him several questions about the brain (which he was delighted to talk about, given the alternative). On the basis of what he had learned in school, he was impressed with the brain. It does "millions of things" he told me, and a person could die if it were seriously damaged. The brain, he solemnly explained, is an extremely important part of your body.

I then asked Max to describe some of the things that the brain does, and he listed seeing, hearing, smelling, and, most of all, thinking. But there were many things that the brain does not do—you use your brain to help go to sleep, but dreaming is not a function of the brain, according to Max. Neither is feeling sad, nor loving his brother. Max said that this is what *he* does, though he admitted that the brain might help him out.

Max has been taught that the brain is important for thinking. But when children learn this, they take "thinking" in the narrow sense, in terms of conscious problem solving and reasoning. If you ask children of this age whether they can go for long periods without doing any thinking at all, they will say yes. The natural conception of the brain by children, even after science education, is that it is a tool we use for certain mental operations. It is a cognitive pros-thesis, added to the soul to increase its computing power.

I doubt that this understanding is much different from that of many adults. Much excitement has been generated by recent stud-ies showing increased neural activity—part of the brain "lighting up" in a scanner—when subjects think about religion, or sex, or race. The details of these findings are plainly relevant for theories of the location and time-course of different mental activities, but people often seem fascinated by the mere fact that the brain is in-volved at all.

For some of us, important psychological traits are seen as related to parts of the body other than the brain. If you tell children about a heart transplant, they sometimes say that this would involve the transfer of traits such as kindness. Some adults would agree. As de-scribed in her book *Change of Heart,* after Claire Sylvia had a heart-lung transplant, she developed a craving for beer and chicken, grew aggressive and confident, and walked with a swagger. She attributed these traits to the properties of her donor, Tim. For what it is worth, her therapist agreed: "I am beginning to believe that some of Tim's essence has transmigrated to Claire."

How does everyday experience change the child's initial belief about the immaterial basis of the soul? If a child's father has a certain ap-pearance on Monday, his appearance is likely to be more or less the same on Tuesday. The child herself will be stuck with the same body through her whole life, and while this body undergoes changes both gradual and abrupt, it will still seem to be the same object.

Furthermore, our relationship to our own body is. . . intimate. This observation troubled Descartes. He was fond of the analogy of soul as pilot and body as vessel. But he was aware that the analogy is imperfect in an important regard. A ship's captain does not experi-ence damage to his ship in anything like the same way that a person experiences pain. Similarly, a ship's captain controls the ship, but our own relationship to the action of our bodies is quite different. It is *closer*. Consider the ruminations of a particularly introspective 13-year-old in Ian McEwan's novel *Atonement*:

> She raised one hand and flexed its fingers and wondered, as she had sometimes before, how this thing, this machine for gripping, this fleshy spider on the end of her arm, came to be hers, entirely at her command. Or did it have some little life of its own? She bent her finger and straightened it. The mystery was in the instant before it moved, the dividing moment between not moving and moving, when her intention took effect. It was like a wave breaking. . . . She brought her forefinger closer to her face and stared at it, urging it to move. It remained still because she was pretending, she was not entirely serious, and because willing to move it, or being about to move it, was not the same as actually moving it. And when she did crook it finally, the action seemed to start in the finger itself, not in some part of her mind. When did it know to move, when did she know how to move it? . . . She knew that behind the smooth continuous fabric was the real self—was it her soul?—which took the decision to cease pretending, and gave the final command.

You do not command your finger to move, or will it to move, or tell it to move. *You just move it.* This is our everyday experience, and it is reasonable to wonder whether, over the course of years, this experience should make the assumption of body/soul duality go away. It should persuade the developing child that we do not *occupy* our bodies; we *are* our bodies.

If our thoughts and actions were in perfect synchrony, then we might really see them as one and the same. But our bodies betray us. We stumble getting up because our foot falls asleep, we drop a plate, spill our drink, and so on. Theologians have not missed this failure of thoughts and actions to fit perfectly. Consider Augustine's famous argument that involuntary sexual arousal and impotence are divine punishments after the Fall. Garry Wills states, "The chanciness of arousal shows the loss of the integrity, the unison, of body and soul." But the unfaithfulness of our bodies does not begin with sexual dysfunction. It is experienced by any baby who howls in frustration at the challenge of learning to crawl.

DEATH

The understanding that people can be the same even after radical transformations of their bodies is only weak evidence for the attribution of souls. After all, houses also retain their identities after centuries of renovations and rebuilding. But we do not think houses have souls.

What is unique to people is the assumption that personhood can survive the destruction of the body. It makes no sense to say that if a fork were destroyed, its "essence" might survive, perhaps showing up in a later existence as a spoon. Forks and spoons do not have essences in that sense and they do not have bodies; they are bodies. But many do believe that when a person dies, the soul leaves the body and goes somewhere: to heaven, to hell, to some unspecified nether world, or into the body of some other creature, human or animal. If I say that I am the reincarnation of the queen of France, you probably won't believe me, but you can understand what I am saying. If you hear about my near-death experience or how I was hypnotically regressed so as to remember my past life, you may be convinced, or unsure, or you might think it is total bunk—but you understand the claims. The existence of research into parapsychology more generally suggests that these claims, regardless of their truth, are understandable even to skeptics.

The relationship between a belief in life after death and our intuitive dualism is complex. One can be a dualist but believe that when the body is gone, the soul goes too. Conversely, one can believe in life after death without being a dualist. You might put your faith in the idea that consciousness arises not from specific brain matter but from the information that the brain encodes. If so, immortality might not be so far away. Ray Kurzweil predicts that by 2040, the technology will be available to upload yourself onto a computer, so that if your body is destroyed, you can be downloaded into a robot or a cloned body. Or you might believe that God will resurrect you physically, including your brain. Indeed, Elaine Pagels notes the central importance the early Christians gave to the fact that when Jesus rose from the dead, it was Jesus' actual physical body. He said, "Handle me and see, for a spirit does not have flesh and bones, as you see that I have." To convince his disciples, he asked for some food and ate it. His body was resurrected, not merely his soul.

Even if one believes that the soul is distinct from the body and survives death, it does not follow that corpses are unimportant. On the contrary, every culture treats dead bodies with some degree of reverence and care. Sometimes they are buried, often with clothes, weapons, and other cherished or useful objects; sometimes they are burned, sometimes eaten. But there is always some proper procedure that must be carried out. Many are horrified at the thought that their bodies, or those of their family or friends, will not get the proper respect.

This anxiety shows up in wartime. People worry about death on the battlefield, but they worry as well about what happens after death. The 1949 Geneva Convention explicitly states that the victors of a battle must "search for the [enemy's] dead and prevent their being despoiled," and ensure that "the dead are honorably interred, if possible according to the rites of the religion to which they belonged." Contemporary military forces will go through great efforts to recover the bodies of fallen comrades, and the desecration of these bodies—as when dead American soldiers were paraded through the streets of Somalia—is met with anguish and rage.

The problem with souls is that they are invisible and intangible. As the philosopher Ludwig Wittgenstein put it, "The human body is the best picture of the human soul." When we wish to commune with the dead, we often go to their grave sites. This is as close as we can get. And to the extent that a soul lives on, it is an act of respect and kindness to care for its most prized possession—and what would that be if not its body? Furthermore, under many religious views, the body must be treated with care in order for the soul to make it safely to its final destination.

WHAT CHILDREN
KNOW ABOUT DEATH

We start off with the two distinct stances, which makes it conceivable to us both that a body can persist without a soul and, vice versa, that a soul can persist without a body. If we were intuitive materialists, believing that consciousness and intelligence are the products of physical processes, the idea of an afterlife would make no sense to us.

The first understanding of death is by means of an analogy with sleep or departure, perhaps because this is how it is explicitly described to children. Grandmother is asleep forever. She has gone to heaven. She has left and will never come back. Children also experience some confusion that probably arises from ambiguities of language. A child might hear that Grandmother is buried in the ground *and* that Grandmother is in heaven. An investigator in 1896 reported the following dialogue with his four-year-old son:

Son: It's only naughty people who are buried, isn't it?
Father: Why?
Son: Because Auntie said all the good people went to heaven.

The psychologist Susan Carey has argued that children are also puzzled as to what sorts of things can be dead. To be dead is not to be alive, but all sorts of things are not alive, including ex-living-things (which corresponds to the adult notion of dead things), but also things that are inanimate, and not real. Not everything that is not dead is alive; not everything that is not alive is dead. Children have problems getting this straight. Carey reports a dialogue with her three-year-old daughter that was prompted by the question "Does your bear have blood and bones inside her?"

> Daughter: No, because she is not a big real person. . . . She can never die—she'll always be alive!
> Mother: Is she alive?
> Daughter: No—she's dead. HOW CAN THAT BE?
> Mother: Is she alive or dead?
> Daughter: Dead.
> Mother: Did she used to be alive?
> Daughter: No, she's middle-sized—in between alive and dead.

Then there is flat-out confusion over the mechanics of what happens when one dies. Carey's daughter asked, "How do dead people go to the bathroom?" and observed, "Maybe they have bathrooms under the ground." When Carey responded that dead people don't have to go to the bathroom because they don't eat or drink, her daughter triumphantly replied, "But they ate or drank before they died—they have to go to the bathroom from just before they died." It is not until somewhere between about five and seven years of age that children show a clear adult understanding of what death is—that it is irreversible and inevitable and means a complete cessation of biological function.

Why do so many people believe in an afterlife? Some conception of life after death is common in every culture, and, to judge from burial artifacts, appears to have existed a very long time ago. There are several explanations for this. Ideas about the afterlife are explicitly taught to people, and socially maintained, in part because they serve the interests of the powerful, who exert social control by means of the carrot of heaven and the stick of hell. Also, many are impressed with what they see as positive evidence for life after death, such as near-death experiences and communication with the departed (recall that about one in six Americans claim to have spoken to the dead).

Furthermore, the notion of oblivion, of a finite life followed by nothingness, is horrifying to many. I would much rather believe that my loved ones are rejoicing in heaven than that they are simply gone, and I have a similar preference with regard to my own fate. Wishful thinking is not in itself an explanation for the existence of a belief. I wish I could fly, but I don't believe that I can fly. But the inability to fly is obvious, while the state of the soul after death is not. For most of human history, there was no scientific reason to doubt that the soul can outlast the body. Because this view is fully conceivable (since we see the soul and the body as separate) and extremely tempting (since we do not want our souls to cease to exist), it is an easy belief to adopt.

Most of all, belief in an afterlife is a natural consequence of our intuitive Cartesian perspective. Consider again Descartes' own intuition that the experience of the body is different from the experience of the self, of the soul. I can imagine my body being destroyed, my brain ceasing to function, my bones turning to dust, but it is harder—some would say impossible—to imagine my self no longer existing. This implies that we should find it easier to understand the cessation of biological function (death of the body) than the cessation of mental function (death of the soul). And it implies that even young children should believe that the soul survives the destruction of the body.

To explore children's beliefs about this, the psychologists Jesse Bering and David Bjorklund told children a story about an alligator and a mouse that ended with the destruction of the mouse: "Uh-oh! Mr. Alligator sees Brown Mouse and is coming to get him!" Children are then shown a picture of the alligator eating the mouse.

"Well, it looks like Brown Mouse got eaten by Mr. Alligator. Brown Mouse is not alive anymore."

Then they asked the children questions about the mouse's biological functioning: "Now that the mouse is no longer alive. . . "

Will he ever need to go to the bathroom?
Do his ears still work?
Does his brain still work?

And they asked about the mouse's mental functioning: "Now that the mouse is no longer alive. . . "

Is he still hungry?
Is he thinking about the alligator?
Does he still want to go home?

The results were striking. When asked about biological properties, four-to-six-year-olds appreciated the effects of death—no need for bathroom breaks, the ears don't work, and neither does the brain. The mouse's body is gone. But when asked about the psychological properties, over half of the children said that they would *continue*—the mouse can experience hunger, thoughts, and desires. The soul survives.

Freud proposed that the "doctrine of the soul" emerged as a solution to the problem of death: if souls exist, then conscious experience need not come to an end. In contrast, I propose that this doctrine exists from the very start. Young children do not know that they will one day die. But once they learn about the inevitable destruction of their body, the notion of an afterlife comes naturally. This is the most important consequence of seeing the world as Descartes did.

8

GODS, SOULS, AND SCIENCE

We firmly believe and profess without qualification that there is only one true God—Creator of all things visible and invisible, spiritual and corporeal. By His almighty power from the very beginning of time, He has created both orders of creatures in the same way out of nothing, the spiritual or angelic world and the corporeal or visible universe. And afterwards He formed the creature man, who in a way belongs to both orders, as he is composed of spirit and body.

> Fourth Lateran Council, 1215; reaffirmed by Pope Pius XII,
> *Humani Generis* (*Of the Human Race*), 1950

There is only one religion, though there are a hundred versions of it.

> —George Bernard Shaw

MOST PEOPLE I KNOW believe in a God who created the universe, performs miracles, and listens to prayers. He is omnipotent and omniscient, possessing infinite kindness, justice, and mercy. But this is because most people I know are Christians or Jews. The Uduk-speaking people of Sudan think that ebony trees overhear the conversations of people who talk beneath them. Pygmies of the Ituri forest in the Democratic Republic of the Congo believe that their entire forest looks after them, and is particularly generous to good people. The Aymara of the Andes describe a mountain as a live body that feeds on the meat of sacrificed animals and, if treated properly, will ensure the fertility of the fields. Mayotte islanders of the Indian Ocean believe in invisible people who take over bodies and have insatiable desires for, of all things, cologne.

What do all of these spiritual entities have in common? Why is it that we come to believe in them? I suggest that many of our religious notions are by-products of a mind that has evolved to think in terms of bodies and souls. I conclude this chapter by turning to the question of whether bodies and souls really exist. How well does our commonsense view of the world mesh with the discoveries of science?

SUPERNATURAL BEINGS

The anthropologist Pascal Boyer has come up with a way to characterize the sorts of entities that appear within religious or supernatural worldviews: supernatural entities represent an optimal compromise between the interesting and the expected.

The criterion of interestingness is obvious: supernatural entities have to be interesting, because if they were not memorable and worth talking about, they would never spread throughout a culture and be sustained over time. Boyer suggests that they become interesting by violating some aspect of our commonsense understanding; they are *counterintuitive*. This is true almost by definition: if a notion did not violate our commonsense understanding of reality, why would we think of it as supernatural in the first place? Ghosts are immaterial people, their immateriality being interesting and easy to remember and worth talking about because it violates our usual experience that people can be seen and touched.

Aside from its counterintuitive, interesting features, however, a supernatural entity's properties have to be just what one would expect for a normal entity. Once you learn that ghosts are immaterial people, you assume that they have beliefs and goals, can understand language and interpret facial expressions, and have normal likes and dislikes—just like normal people. If you hear about conscious trees, you can safely assume that aside from possessing consciousness, everything else that is normally true of trees applies: they grow and eventually die, provide shade, have leaves, are solid, are visible, do not fly, and so on. If an entity were too weird, it would be confusing and difficult to recall, and hence would not be sustained within a culture.

Boyer's hypothesis has led him to create what he calls the *Catalogue of Supernatural Templates*:

> Persons can be represented as having counterintuitive physical properties (e.g., ghosts or gods), counterintuitive biology (many gods who neither grow or die) or counterintuitive psychological properties (unblocked perception or prescience). Animals too can have all these properties. Tools and other artifacts can be represented as having biological properties (some statues bleed) or psychological ones (they hear what you say). Browsing through volumes of mythology, fantastic tales, anecdotes, cartoons, religious writings and science fiction, you will get an extraordinary variety of different *concepts,* but you will also find that the number of *templates* is very limited and in fact contained in the short list above.

If we stopped here, it would not be very satisfying. After being told about a certain belief, any clever person could, after the fact, tell a story how it is an optimal compromise between the interesting and expected. Can this theory of supernatural templates be used to make predictions? To find out, Boyer, in collaboration with the psychologist Justin Barrett, engaged in some "experimental theology," using methods from experimental psychology to explore the nature of religious belief.

Their experiments tested the prediction that people will find it easiest to remember novel entities that profoundly violate a single expectation of common sense, such as a man who walks though walls or a table that feels sad. Being merely unusual, such as having six fingers, is not enough. Boyer and Barrett also predicted that these entities characterized by singular violations are easier to remember than those that have multiple violations, such as a statue that hears what you say (an artifact with psychological properties) *and* disappears every now and then (a violation of physics).

They tested not just the usual populations of college undergraduates, but also the Fang people of West Africa (both in a large city and in villages in the forest) and Tibetan monks in Nepal. In all cases, the results fit their predictions. The easiest supernatural entity to remember violates exactly one fundamental property.

There is something else that the notions we find in religion and everything listed in Boyer's catalogue have in common. All of these supernatural notions involve the attribution of mental states.

This is most obvious for ghosts and gods, but it holds as well for anomalies such as hungry mountains and bleeding statues. They are not merely objects and artifacts with bizarre biological properties; they also have psychological properties such as beliefs and desires. Other anomalies, such as virgin birth, the transformation of water into wine, and the parting of the Red Sea, are not themselves intentional entities, but they are associated with souls in that they are seen as the consequence of intentional action, as miracles that occur through the wishes of a divine creature.

With this in mind, here is my own method for creating a supernatural being:

1. Start with the notion of an immaterial soul.
2. Embody or modify it in an unusual way.
3. Stir in interesting details.

A soul can exist without a body, as a spirit, ghost, or deity. Or a soul might exist in an unusual body, such as a mountain or a tree, or in a body that belongs to someone else, as when a person is possessed. Souls can leave the body through dreams, trances, and death. Souls might control entities from a distance, and can have unusual powers of perception, knowledge, or causation. The most extreme example of this is the Judeo-Christian God. But none of this violates our foundational understanding of how souls work. No religion has ever posited supernatural beings who get very angry when you do what they want, or who always do the opposite of what they intend to do.

It is worth keeping in mind that religion is not the only source of counterintuitive beliefs. Contemporary scientific theories of the origin of the universe, the nature of matter, and the structure of thought are a lot more bizarre than anything you will find in the Bible, the Koran, or the Tibetan Book of the Dead. Just focusing on the domain of psychology, consider that some neuroscientists think that each hemisphere of the brain is actually a distinct person. Some philosophers think that consciousness is a basic property of the universe, existing in some limited degree even in rocks and stars. Some computer scientists say that machines are, or can be, conscious. And the reigning theory in the cognitive sciences—what the biologist Francis Crick called "the astonishing hypothesis"—is that our selves are the results of brain processes. This is profoundly counterintuitive.

When distinguishing between science and religion, to look for a difference in the *content* of beliefs is the wrong approach. Better instead to examine the *process* through which these beliefs come about, and the social conditions under which they are maintained and modified. If a person believes in ghosts because she has been persuaded by empirical evidence and is willing to test her views and possibly reject them on the basis of the data, this is a scientific hypothesis. To the extent that her belief is rooted in faith and cannot be swayed by evidence, it is religion.

GOD

The psychologists Justin Barrett and Frank Keil coined the term "theological correctness" to draw attention to the distinction between theological notions endorsed by religious authorities (which people might explicitly cite if asked) and beliefs that arise from people's intuitions. The former can be out of sync with the latter. In 1999, Pope John Paul II stated that heaven and hell are not places, but instead refer to different states of life, to whether or not one is in relation to God. Many Catholics were shocked at this statement. Some wrote letters to newspapers complaining that the aged pope must have lost his mind. These Catholics may reluctantly come to accept this theologically correct interpretation, but they may also continue to reflexively think of heaven and hell as they did before the pope's proclamation: places where souls reside.

The same sort of tension might exist between theologically correct and intuitive notions of God. If you were to ask most Jews or Christians what God is, they would describe Him as an all-knowing and all-powerful deity. This is the theologically correct view. But our intuitive understanding might be tainted by the biases we have toward construing souls—even those we see as belonging to deities—in our own image. This is not a new idea: As Voltaire said, God created man in His own image and man promptly returned the compliment.

Indeed, a singular omniscient, omnipotent, immortal benign god is an unusual entity to believe in. Buddhism lacks any such deity.

Other religions have a multitude of spirits, some of which are mean and stupid. In Siberia, metaphorical language is used when discussing important matters, so as to confound literal-minded spirits. In parts of Africa, it is good manners when visiting friends and relatives to tell them how ugly and unpleasant their children are—so that witches, who are looking for good children to harm, will lose interest and look elsewhere.

Certainly the God of the Old Testament had human qualities. As He Himself puts it: "For you should worship no other god, because the LORD, whose name is Jealous, is a jealous God." There is a fine humanness in the Lord's bitterness at the ungratefulness of the Israelis: "How long will this people despise me? And how long will they not believe in me, in spite of all the signs which I have wrought among them? I will strike them with the pestilence and disinherit them." There are many who see every calamity in modern times, from the Holocaust to the AIDS virus to the loss of a pivotal football game, as the expression of God's anger or disappointment.

People insist that God is nonphysical, formless, and omnipresent, but they also admit to seeing Him in more concrete forms, often as an old man living in the sky. Barrett and Keil explored this tension in a series of experiments with adults from both the United States and India. When explicitly asked about their religious beliefs, these adults said that God has no physical or spatial properties, can know and attend everything at once, and is omnipotent. Then Barrett and Keil gave them a series of stories about God. (For the Hindu subjects, "God" was replaced by Shiva, Krishna, Brahman, or Vishnu.) One story went like this:

A boy was swimming alone in a swift and rocky river. The boy got his left leg caught between two large, gray rocks and couldn't get out. Branches of trees kept bumping into him as they hurried past. He thought he was going to drown and so he began to struggle and

pray. Though God was answering another prayer in another part of
the world when the boy started praying, before long God responded
by pushing one of the rocks so the boy could get his leg out. They
boy struggled to the riverbank, and fell over exhausted.

When later asked about this story, people often say that it explicitly said that God *first* had to finish answering the first prayer and
once he was finished went on to save the boy's life. But the story actually doesn't specify a timeline—and if people believed that God
could perform an infinite number of tasks at once, this scheduling
pileup should not occur. Barrett and Keil argue that people's commonsense understanding distorts their memory in an anthropo-
morphic direction and they tend to treat God as if He had the
limitations of a person. Other studies found that Catholics and
Protestants who go to churches with images of Jesus, the Holy
Spirit, or God were more likely to interpret the story this way, suggesting that exposure to religious images plays some role in encour-
aging anthropomorphism.

I have found that some people find such research somehow disturbing, even sacrilegious, so I want to end this section with two reassuring points. First, the questions of what people think about God
and how they come to have these beliefs are logically separate from
the question of whether God exists. One does not have to be an
atheist to study religious thought. If God does exist, there still remains the psychological question of how we understand Him. Second, results such as Barrett and Keil's should not be taken as
showing that people "really" believe that God is a person. Just because a belief is theologically correct and possibly not intuitive does
not mean that it cannot be sincere. What the research cited above
suggests is that there are certain natural ways of thinking about
God, and about souls in general, and these clash with the tenets of

certain religions. Those who are devout might view this as confirming that the human mind is not adequate to appreciate the nature of God. Those who adopt a more secular perspective might take it as a demonstration of how culture can create and sustain beliefs that mesh poorly with commonsense intuitions.

DO CHILDREN BELIEVE IN MAGIC?

Developmental psychologists such as Jean Piaget have proposed that children start off with a mind unconstrained by logic and rationality, making them particularly willing to believe in supernatural entities and events. These psychologists say that children are prone to magical thought.

Children do seem to accept weird things. When Max was four years old, I told him a story about how you could step into his closet and it would magically take you back through time to the land of dinosaurs. He took me seriously, insisted that we actually try it out, and was annoyed when it did not work. The psychologist Eugene Subbotsky showed four-to-six-year-olds a magic box that, he said, turned drawings into real objects if you said the magic words "alpha beta gamma." When the experimenter left them alone in the room with the box and a set of drawings, almost all of the children tried the machine out. They put drawings in the box, said "alpha beta gamma," and looked disappointed when nothing happened. In another study, Subbotsky told children about a magic potion that makes children younger and then left them alone with the potion, saying, "Now you can try the water if you want. I want to see if it works. But if you do not want to try—it is up to you." Most refused to drink the water. Other researchers have found that when young children are asked to imagine that a box contains a monster who likes to bite fingers, they will keep away from it.

But what do these findings really show? After all, children are exposed to technological wonders like remote-control cars, microwave ovens, and video cameras. How could they know that the technology for time travel, transforming drawings into objects, and age regression is not quite there yet? Is a device that turns drawings into real things really any weirder than such real-world machines as a robot vehicle that flies to Mars? Many children wonder if the people on television can see them. But of course there *are* such things as video cameras; such children are not displaying magical thought, they are just showing some healthy paranoia.

Finally, children do not really think things that they imagine are real. If you ask children to imagine that a pencil is in a box and then someone comes in and asks if anyone knows where a pencil is, children do not direct the person to the box. In fact, young children actually seem to have the world of make-believe and real-life pretty well worked out. Even three-year-olds are clear that ghosts, monsters, and witches are "make-believe" and dogs, houses, and bears are "real-life." Most likely they avoid the finger-biting monster for the same reason that adults cringe in horror movies. People of all ages can be affected by fantasy and illusion. Adults will often refuse to eat a turd-shaped block of fudge or drink a glass with "cyanide" written on it, even if they themselves had just filled it with water. In an unpublished study conducted by Jonathan Haidt, college students who insisted that they were atheists were asked to write and sign a contract selling their soul to the devil; many refused.

Adults sometimes respond to fictional characters as if they were real people. The actor Robert Young, who played the lead role in the television show *Marcus Welby, M.D.,* reported getting thousands of letters each week asking for medical advice; he later exploited this confusion by appearing in commercials to tout the health benefits of Sanka decaffeinated coffee. Soap-opera fans react strongly to their beloved and hated characters, and when Charles Dickens had his character Little Nell die, he was deluged with enraged letters. It is not clear what is going on here. Does an adult sitting down to write Marcus Welby about the pain in his foot really know, at some level, that Welby is just a fictional character? Is this an elaborate form of pretense? Is it similar to a child chasing an imaginary dog around the house? Or is there some real confusion? In any case, it is plain that illusion does have a visceral effect on adults as well as children.

Children do sometimes create beings that do not really exist. The psychologist Marjorie Taylor reports that about half of the young children she studied had imaginary companions. One four-year-old told Taylor about two invisible birds, one male (named Nutsy), the other female (also named Nutsy). They were raucous and clumsy, and talked incessantly. Other imaginary companions reported by parents and investigators include a chest of drawers; a giant who steps out of walls to chop off children's hands; a pair of creatures named Honia (who is full of honey) and Jellia (who is full of jelly); two creatures named Phena and Barbara Tall (created by a girl whose father was on medication); a pretend friend named Throat who lives in the child's throat; and Station Pheta, who has big beady eyes and a big blue head and hunts for sea anemones and dinosaurs at the beach.

These creations can offer companionship, alleviate loneliness, allow for the development of rich and enjoyable fantasies, and provide a safe means of communicating to others. (When Jean Piaget's daughter Jacqueline was angry with him, she would express this anger by talking about the father of her imaginary companion: "Marecage has a horrid father. . . . Her mother chose badly.")

Do these imaginary companions show that children have problems distinguishing fantasy from reality? Only if children do not know that they are imaginary. Taylor collected evidence on this issue by asking children questions about the properties of imaginary and real things. She noted that a particularly clear sign of their sophistication was that, at some point in the interview, after being asked several questions about their companions, the children would often gently tell the psychologists something like "It's just pretend, you know."

WHAT DO
CHILDREN KNOW ABOUT GOD?

The evidence from developmental psychology suggests that there is nothing particularly magical about children's style of thought. How then do they cope with the religious ideas that they get from the culture?

Some of these ideas are confusing. The psychologist Jacqueline Woolley finds that children take a while to understand what prayer is and how it works. In fact, they find the notion of "wishing," which is a nonreligious concept, much easier to grasp. Children younger than five do not understand that God is involved in prayer, and fail to appreciate that it is the interaction between God and thoughts that is the point of prayer.

What about children's thoughts about God? For many children, belief in God is initially on a par with a belief in the Tooth Fairy and Santa Claus. Some children state that God and Santa Claus live close to each other and that they are friends, or that God instructs Santa about whom to give presents to. For this reason, many fundamentalist parents are uncomfortable with myths such as Santa Claus. They feel that once their children learn that Santa Claus does not exist—and that they have been lied to about this—they might question what they have been told about God and Jesus. These parents are worrying too much; very few children lose their belief in God when they learn about Santa. But this is only because the existence of God continues to be established socially.

Freud and Piaget both proposed that children might start off seeing God as a person, as a powerful and protective adult, and this has been supported. Children describe God as having a face, a body, and a voice. If you ask three-year-olds questions about the properties of God and about the properties of their best friend, they do not make any systematic distinction between the two. The mature appreciation that, unlike a person, God is omniscient and that God is unchanging does not show up until about the age of five, and even some five-year-olds are a bit fuzzy. God might know what is inside a closed box "because he does magic," but he would be confused if the wrapping does not match what is inside. God will never die, but he was once a baby and grew "because he ate a lot."

This notion of a human-like God is even encouraged by some parents, who tell their children that God will be pleased or angry—or even hurt—by their behaviors. Sometimes they also appeal to the limitations of God as a response to children's worries about the problem of evil. An illustrative anecdote comes from a recent *New York Times* article: After a young girl was murdered by a serial killer in California, another girl asked, "Mommy, why didn't God help her?" Her mother told her that "there are a lot of crazy people out there and he can't watch over all of them at the same time."

For all of us, but particularly for children, there is a pull toward the human, a natural assumption that other entities will share our cognitive powers and our bodily constraints. Many four-year-olds say a tulip can feel happy and can feel pain, and they think that elephants, snakes, ants, and even trees have beliefs. Our capacity for understanding intention has evolved to deal with people, and so we tend to extend a people-like analysis even to creatures whose powers are much weaker (tulips) or stronger (God).

This leads to a surprising prediction. Individuals with autism should not be as prone to anthropomorphize God, since they lack the same intention-based mode of interpretation. Jesse Bering has recently summarized the evidence that bears on this issue, and observes that autobiographical accounts by high-functioning individuals with

autism suggest that their notions of God are unusual in just this regard. Edgar Schneider, in his book *Discovering My Autism*, insisted
that "my belief in the existence of a supreme intelligence (or, if you
will, a God) is based on scientific factors," and he noted that he felt
no emotional and personal feelings about such a being. Temple
Grandin, who is well known for her insights into what it means to be
autistic, has written: "In high school I came to the conclusion that
God was an ordering force that was in everything. . . . In nature, particles are entangled with millions of other particles, all interacting
with each other. One could speculate that the entanglement of these
particles could create a kind of consciousness for the universe. That
is my current concept of God."

The evidence suggests that children are not born with any capacities or dispositions that are special to religious ideas. There is no
religion module or innate notion of God, nothing akin to the "language organ" proposed by Noam Chomsky or the moral emotions
discussed in the previous chapters. Children are highly prone to attribute thoughts, emotions, and goals; as a result, it is natural for
them to make sense of entities such as gods, spirits, and ghosts. But
children do not generate these entities from nothing; they are con-
sumers of religious ideas, not producers.

BODY AND SOUL

It would be irresponsible to end a book about how children and
adults think about bodies and souls without discussing whether
there really are bodies and souls. When we see the world in this way,
are we right?

It might be tempting to conclude that bodies and souls must exist
because a belief in them is innate, shaped by natural selection. But
this is a weak argument. The driving force behind natural selection
is survival and reproduction, not truth. All other things being equal,

it is better for an animal to believe true things than false things; accurate perception is better than hallucination. But sometimes all other things are not equal. We have some innate fear of snakes, but this does not mean that snakes are a real hazard in the world we now live in (they are not); we are repelled by the smell of dung, but this does not mean that dung has an objective quality of being repellent (it does not—dung beetles like it just fine). If "innate" meant "true," we would not need to do physics; we could get the scoop on the universe just by studying babies.

On the other extreme, one might argue that bodies and souls do not exist because the only proper description of the world is given in the language of physics. Because of this, there are no chairs, clocks, forks, fish, or people. All that really exists is elementary forces, quarks, leptons, and whatever else that physicists discover.

But this is far too minimalist a perspective. The natural sciences such as chemistry, biology, and geology explain lawful generalizations at levels above that of physics, some of them involving real-world objects. The philosopher Hilary Putnam makes the point that nothing at the level of physics can explain why a square peg cannot fit in a round hole. If you want to explain this you need to be able to talk about pegs and holes. There is no reason to doubt that the world really does contain *bodies:* material entities that move on continuous paths through time and space, that are solid, and that affect one another though contact. Babies are right, then, to believe that the world contains such entities. This conception is incomplete, of course—at a different level, such objects are actually composed of tiny particles whizzing through empty space. But incomplete is not the same as mistaken.

What about souls? At the core of our attribution of souls is a belief in the existence of entities with mental lives. Their actions are not to be explained in terms of brute physical forces, the way one would understand the movement of a rock or a baseball, but are instead the results of what they know and what they desire. If you see a ball rolling toward a door, you assume that it is moving because some force pushed it, but if you see a person moving toward a door, you assume that he or she has a reason for doing so.

It is reassuring how much of this belief system has been supported by the sciences of the mind. Radical behaviorists once ridiculed the notion of internal mental processes. Gilbert Ryle famously called it "the doctrine of the Ghost in the Machine." But with the invention of the computer, the doctrine is not very funny anymore. We know now that physical objects can store information, draw inferences, use symbols, and so on. These work not through magic, but through principles discovered by mathematicians like Alan Turing and Alonzo Church, who explored how purely physical devices can store information and manipulate this information in a rational way. These discoveries made possible the discipline of cognitive psychology, which has had impressive success explaining capacities such as language and perception. This in turn has led to cognitive neuroscience, which explores the precise means by which the brain encodes and uses information.

Common sense also tells us that there are emotions such as anger, joy, disgust, and fear; that we have drives pushing us toward food, drink, sex, companionship; that we love our children and hate those who treat us shabbily. Nothing from neuroscience, evolutionary biology, or developmental psychology provides any reason to doubt that this is true. Emotions are real, and they drive our actions in pretty much the way that we naturally assume that they do.

This is the good news.

Some scholars think it is all good news. Science does not conflict with common sense, and does not conflict with religion. Stephen Jay Gould argued that both science and religion have their own independent realms: "Science covers the empirical realm: what the universe is made of (fact) and why does it work this way (theory). Religion extends over questions of ultimate meaning and moral value."

Gould may well be right about the scope of science, but he is wrong about religion. To say that religion does not extend over the domain of fact is true only of the most toothless and secularized belief systems, such as certain cheerful New Age movements. Real religions posit survival of memories and desires after death and divine interventions that split seas and defeat armies. They make substantive empirical claims about the origin of the universe, the Earth, animals, and especially humans. They take positions about the curative powers of prayer, about the existence of entities such as angels and demons, and so on. These are substantive claims about what the world is made of and why it works the way it does. And some of these claims have to do with the nature of bodies and souls.

Don't take my word for it. In 1996, the pope accepted Darwin's theory of evolution as applying to nonhumans, and perhaps to human bodies, but he added the following qualification:

> If the human body takes its origin from pre-existent living matter, the spiritual soul is immediately created by God. . . . Consequently, theories of evolution which, in accordance with the philosophies inspiring them, consider the spirits as emerging from the forces of living matter or as a mere epiphenomenon of this matter, are incompatible with the truth about man.

This is the bad news. Science tells us that mental life is the product of the mind; it *does* emerge from living matter. All thought is the result of biochemical processes, and damage to the brain leads to mental impairments, destroying capacities as central to our humanity as self-control, the ability to reason, and our capacity for love. There may well be a spiritual soul, but it is not distinct from the forces of matter.

Some scholars are optimistic about what cognitive science tells us about ourselves. In *The Blank Slate,* Steven Pinker concludes that acknowledging certain facts about human nature, including the fact that there is no such thing as an immaterial soul, does not have the negative consequences many people think it does. On the contrary, it supports some of the values that we hold most dear. And Owen Flanagan's *The Problem of the Soul* is written with the goal of showing that a scientific conception of human nature can "retain what is beautiful, true, and inspiring in the humanistic image."

I am optimistic too. I think there is nothing from the study of evolution and psychology that leads us to doubt the most important and worthwhile aspects of our selves. Richard Dawkins said that only since Darwin is it possible to be an intellectually fulfilled atheist. Similarly, I think that only now, with the converging work of philosophers, psychologists, and evolutionary theorists, is it possible to be a morally optimistic materialist.

But I do not underestimate the clash between the scientific view of mental functioning and the commonsense one. Cognitive scientists believe that emotions, memories, and consciousness are the result of physical processes. Common sense tells us that our mental life is the product of an immaterial soul, and this intuition gives rise to the deeply reassuring idea that the soul can survive the destruction of the body and brain. A belief in the physical basis of thought is very much a minority viewpoint.

Things are just beginning to heat up. When people hear about research into the neural basis of thought, they learn about specific findings: this part of the brain is involved in risk taking, that part is active when someone thinks about music, and so on. But the bigger picture, the material basis of thought, is not yet generally appreciated, and it is interesting to ponder how people will react when it is. (We are seeing the first signs now, much of it in the recent work of novelists such as Jonathan Franzen, David Lodge, and Ian McEwan.)

It might be that nonspecialists will learn to live with the fact that our intuitions about the self are mistaken, just as those of us who are not physicists have come to accept that apparently solid objects are composed of tiny moving particles.

This will not be easy. The notion that our souls are flesh is profoundly troubling. The same sorts of controversies that have raged over the study and teaching of evolution in the last hundred years are likely to erupt in the cognitive sciences in the years to come. We are in for some interesting times.

NOTES

PREFACE

xi Darwin on uniquely human traits: Darwin 1998 [1872], 1874; see also Cronin 1992.

xii Cartesian dualism: Descartes 1641; see Flanagan 1984 for discussion.

xii Descartes' robot baby: Gaukroger 1995; Reé 2002; Wood 2002.

CHAPTER 1: MINDREADERS

3 Master gambler: Alvarez 2001, 67.

6 What objects are: Spelke 1994; Spelke et al. 1993.

6 Pulling as a test for objects: Pinker 1997.

7 Dumb babies: *The Onion*, 21 May 1997.

7 A perfect idiot: Cited in Rochat 2001, 5.

8 Out of sight, out of mind: Piaget 1954.

9 Problems with coordinated action: Diamond 1991.

10 Missing part of stick: Kellman and Spelke 1983.

10 Newborn chicks: Regolin and Vallortigara 1995.

10 Baby arithmetic: Wynn 1992; **review of replications:** Wynn 2000; **mathematical monkeys:** Hauser, MacNeilage, and Ware 1996; **arithmetical dogs:** West and Young 2002.

11 Baby understanding of . . . cohesion: Xu, Carey, and Welsh 1999; **continuity:** Spelke, Phillips, and Woodward 1995; **solidity:** Baillargeon, Spelke, and Wasserman 1985; **contact:** Spelke, Phillips, and Woodward 1995.

12 Magical appearance: Wynn and Chiang 1998.

12 The developing understanding of gravity: Baillargeon 2002 (figure 1.2 based on her figure 3.3).

14 Curved motion: McCloskey, Caramazza, and Green 1980; Proffitt and Gilden 1989.

14 Water out of curved tube: Kaiser, Jonides, and Alexander 1986.

14 Response to a still-face: Tronick et al. 1978.

15 Baby video-conferencing: Field et al. 1986; Murray and Trevarthen 1985.

15 **Preference for faces:** Slater and Quinn 2001.

15 **Preference for mom's face:** Field et al. 1984.

15 **Happy vs. sad faces:** Walker-Andrews 1997.

15 **Baby imitation:** Meltzoff and Moore 1977, 1983.

15 **Hands and sticks:** Woodward 1998.

15 **Pointing and looking:** Bretherton 1992; Corkum and Moore 1995; Hobson 2002.

15 **Sensitivity to others' emotions when exploring:** Campos and Stenberg 1981.

16 **Chimpanzee pointing:** Call and Tomasello 1994; Povinelli et al. 1997.

16 **Humans vs. chimpanzees at social reasoning:** Tomasello 1998; Tomasello, Call, and Hare 2003; Povinelli and Vonk 2003.

16 **Smart doggie:** Hare et al. 2002.

17 **Simple movie:** Heider and Simmel 1944; **cross-cultural data:** Morris and Peng 1994; **moving groups:** Bloom and Veres 1999.

17 **Anthropomorphism:** Guthrie 1993.

17 **Trigger-happy babies:** Bertenthal et al. 1995; Fox and McDaniel 1982; Rochat, Morgan, and Carpenter 1997.

18 **Babies treat animated characters as if they have mental states:** Gergely et al. 1995; Premack and Premack 1997; see also Johnson, Slaughter, and Carey 1998 for babies' responses to robots.

18 **Good triangle; bad square!:** Kuhlmeier, Wynn, and Bloom, 2003.

18 **One-year-olds understand that adults like broccoli:** Repacholi and Gopnik 1997.

19 **Talking about mental states:** From Bartsch and Wellman 1995, 114, 39, 112.

20 **False-belief task:** The idea is from Dennett 1978; the first experiment was done by Wimmer and Perner 1983; the actual scenario described here is from Baron-Cohen, Leslie, and Frith 1985.

21 **Arguments that children lack a mature understanding of other minds:** See, for instance, Gopnik 1993a; Perner, Leekam, and Wimmer 1987; Wellman, Cross, and Watson 2001.

21 **Arguments that false belief reasoning is hard, even for adults:** See, for instance, Bloom and German 2000; Fodor 1992; Leslie 1987, 1994a, 1994b.

21 **Problems with double bookkeeping outside the domain of beliefs:** Roth and Leslie 1998.

22 **Explaining children's failures as exaggerated version of adult biases:** Birch and Bloom, 2003, under review.

22 **Adults expect others to share their beliefs:** Kelley and Jacoby 1996; Keysar 1994; Wilson and Brekke 1994.

23 **Cross-cultural differences in understanding of other minds:** D'Andrade 1987; Geertz 1983; Lillard 1998; Nisbett et al. 2001.

23 **Keeping the truth from children:** Postman 1982.

24 **Neglect and Balint syndrome:** Rafal 1997, 1998.

25 **Autism:** See Happé 1996 for review.

25 **Autistic children without futures:** Sacks 1995, 246.

26 **Trying to reach autistic children:** Hornby 2000, xiii-xiv.

27 **The cruelest of mothers:** Gopnik, Meltzoff, and Kuhl 1999, 55.

27 **"Mindblindness" theory of autism:** Baron-Cohen, Leslie, and Frith 1985; see also Baron-Cohen 1995.

27 **Being autistic:** Gopnik 1993b.

28 **Autistic children failing false-belief tasks:** Baron-Cohen et al. 1985.

28 **Autistic children not being drawn to faces:** Dawson et al. 1998.

28 **Scary robot:** Sigman et al. 1992.

28 **Hammer on thumb:** Charman et al. 1997.

29 **A funny noise:** From Sacks 1995, 269.

29 **An anthropologist on Mars:** Sacks 1995.

29 **Autistic descriptions of animations:** Klin 2000.

29 **Virginia Woolf:** Klin et al. 2002.

29 **Faces as objects:** Schultz et al. 2000.

30 **The problem with men:** Baron-Cohen 2002.

32 **Skeptics about evolution:** Wallace 1889, cited by Cronin 1992, 354; Polkinghorne 1999, 2–3; the pope, cited by Pinker 2002, 186–187.

32 **Darwin vs. Wallace:** See Cronin 1992.

33 **Exaptations:** Gould and Vrba 1982; **and spandrels:** Gould and Lewontin 1979.

34 **The enhancing power of language:** Dennett 1996, 17. For similar proposals, see Bloom 1994; Carey 2004; Carruthers 1996; Spelke 2003; Vygotsky 1962. For discussion of the limits of language see Bloom 2000; Bloom and Keil 2001; Pinker 1994.

CHAPTER 2: ARTIFACTS

37 **Detachment of autism:** Kanner 1943, 250.

38 **Names for everything:** Locke 1947 [1690].

38 **Funes:** Borges 1964, 63.

39 **Why do we have categories?:** Locke 1947 [1690], 14–15.

40 **A kind of mental glue:** Murphy 2002, 1 and 3.

42 **Objects are not randomly distributed:** Pinker and Bloom 1990.

42 **Not dull catalogues:** Gould 1989, 98; see also Murphy and Medin 1985.

43 **Borges's rumpled list:** Ackerman 2001, 21.

43 **Ways of dying:** Cited by Bowker and Star 1999.

44 **All that glitters is not gold:** See Bloom 2000; Gelman 2003; Pinker 1994.

45 **Gorillae:** Hubbell 2001, 31–32.

46 **Get real:** This heading is cribbed from Dennett 1994.

46 **Locke on essences:** Locke 1947 [1690], 26.

46 **Essentialism:** For philosophical foundations, see Kripke 1971, 1980; Putnam 1973, 1975a; see Medin and Ortony 1989 for the notion of "psychological essentialism," which is the version proposed here.

46 **Children as essentialists:** See Gelman 2003 for review.

46 **Baby-generalizations:** Baldwin, Markman, and Melartin 1993.

46 **Appearance vs. essence in generalization:** Gelman and Markman 1986, 1987.

47 **Dog mutilation:** Gelman and Wellman 1991.

47 **Common name for shared internal stuff:** Diesendruck, Gelman, and Lebowitz 1998.

47 **Transformations:** Keil 1989.

47 **Talking to children about essences:** Gelman 2003; Heath 1986.

48 **Essentialism is universal:** For example, Atran 1998; Diesendruck 2001; Walker 1992; see Gelman 2003 for review.

48 **Essentialism is adaptive:** Bloom 2000; Kornblith 1993; Pinker 1997.

48 **Cancer:** Ahn 2002.

49 **Essentialism Lite:** Bloom 2000.

49 **Escaping from essentialism:** Mayr 1982, 87; see also Dupré 1993; Hull 1965; Mayr 1991; Sober 1994.

49 **Races as extended families:** Pinker 2002.

50 **No such thing as race:** Cosmides, Tooby, and Kurzban 2003; Lewontin 1972; Pinker 2002; Templeton 1998.

50 **Polling data on genetic similarity:** Jayaratne 2001, cited by Gelman 2003, 430.

50 **The facts of genetic similarity:** Cosmides et al. 2003.

51 **Racial essentialism in young children:** Hirschfeld 1996.

51 **A deeply-rooted bad idea:** Hirschfeld 1996, xi.

51 **The things they carried:** O'Brien 1990, 2.

52 **20,000 everyday artifacts:** Norman 1989.

52 **Marx's astonishment:** Basalla 1988.

52 **Wheat, corn, cats, dogs:** Hubbell 2001.

53 **Get a cow:** Bryson 1992.

54 **No such thing as a tree:** Malt 1991.

54 **Fruit or vegetable?:** Willett 2001, 115.

54 **Appearance not enough for artifact categorization:** Bloom 1996, 1998, 2000.

55 **Essentialism for artifacts too:** Bloom 1996, 1998, 2000; Medin 1989; Putnam 1975a.

56 **No doubt about an axe:** Dennett 1990.

56 **Artifact studies with children:** Diesendruck, Markson, and Bloom 2003; Gelman and Bloom 2000; Gutheil et al. in press; Kemler-Nelson 1999; Kemler-Nelson et al. 1995, 2000a, 2000b; Ward et al. 1991.

58 **Genesis and the importance of language:** Macnamara 1982.

58 **The physical process of divine creation:** Kelemen 1996.

58 **Why do we believe?:** Shermer 2000.

58 **Cicero's argument from design:** Quoted in Kelemen 1996.

58 **There must be a designer:** Paley 1828, quoted in Dawkins 1986, 4.

59 **Paley's influence on Darwin:** Dawkins 1986.

59 **The unlikely universe:** Quoted in Shermer 2003.

60 **Hume's skepticism:** Quoted in Kelemen 1996.

60 **Augustine on flatulence:** Wills 1999.

60 **Canadian poll:** From Shermer 2000.

60 **Creationism is resistant to formal instruction:** Almquist and Cronin 1988; Evans 2001.

60 **Misunderstanding Darwinism:** Dawkins 1986, xv.

61 **Artificialists:** Piaget 1929.

61 **Children know that people do not make natural things:** Evans et al. 1996; Gelman and Kremer 1991.

62 **Teleology in children and adults:** Kelemen 1999a, 1999b, 1999c.

62 **Children as creationists:** Evans 1997, 2000.

63 **Keeping quiet about Darwin:** Cited in Humphrey 1996, 7.

CHAPTER 3: ANXIOUS OBJECTS

65 **Pictures and tears:** Elkins 2001.

66 **Reactions of shock and disgust:** Elkins 2001.

66 **Anxious objects:** Rosenberg 1973.

66 **Examples of anxious objects:** Some of these are from Warburton 2003.

67 **Serge vs. Marc on modern art:** Reza 1996, 3 and 15.

68 **Art and status:** Pinker 1997, 522; see also Pinker 2002; Wolfe 1975.

69 **Babies, dolls, and pictures:** DeLoache, Strauss, and Maynard 1979.

69 **Deprived child:** Hochberg and Brooks 1962; see also Ekman and Friesen 1975 for cross-cultural evidence.

70 **Masquerade Ball:** Koestler 1964.

70 **Weird behavior with pictures:** Ninio and Bruner 1978; Perner 1991; Werner and Kaplan 1963.

70 **Grabbing at pictures across cultures:** DeLoache et al. 1998.

71 **How infants react when they reach for a picture:** DeLoache et al. 1998.

71 **Crying from disappointment:** Elkins 2001, 53.

72 **Picture interpretation in young children:** Preissler 2003; Preissler and Carey (under review).

72 **Weird mistakes with pictures:** Beilin and Pearlman 1991; Thomas, Nye, and Robinson 1994.

72 **Doubts that older children really are confused about pictures:** Bloom 2000.

73 **Picasso's postcard:** Danto 1986.

73 **Mortal terror:** Freeman 1991.

73 **Learning how to read a representation:** Ittelson 1996.

73 **Problems with dual representations:** DeLoache 1995; DeLoache and Burns 1994; DeLoache, Miller, and Rosengren 1997.

73 **Dolls in sexual abuse cases:** DeLoache and Marzolf 1995.

74 **Confusions about time:** Friedman 1990.

74 **Art as human universal:** Brown 1991; Dissanayake 1992.

74 **Parallels between child art and adult art:** Gardner 1980, 2–5.

75 **Are children creating representations?** Gardner 1980, 46–47; see also Cox 1992; Freeman 1991; Golomb 1993.

76 **Little Prince:** Saint-Exupéry 1943, 2.

76 Naming based on size and oddity: Bloom and Markson 1998.

77 Mommy and Daddy: Kagan 1981.

77 Fork and spoon: Bloom and Markson 1997.

78 Lollipop and balloon: Bloom and Markson 1998.

78 Picture naming and autism: Preissler 2003; Bloom et al. (under review).

81 Attempts to define art: Davies 1991.

81 The art of Heliogabulus: Lyas 1997.

82 Art is whatever people say it is: For discussion see Danto 1964, 1981; Dickie 1984.

82 Art as intended for an audience: Dickie 1984; Fodor 1993.

83 Art as intended to be art: Levinson 1979, 1989, 1993.

84 What do children see as art? Gelman 2003; Gelman and Ebeling 1998.

86 Chess set: Haugeland 1993.

86 Toys: Woolley and Wellman 1990.

87 Why do visual patterns look good? Marr 1982; Pinker 1997; Ramachandran and Hirstein 1999; Shepard 1990.

87 The beauty of Piss Christ: Julius 2002, 15; Menand 2002, 101.

88 Mapplethorpe's innocent appeal to formalism: Julius 2002.

88 Baffled about art: Sheets 2000.

88 The story of van Meegeren: Werness 1983; Dutton 1983a.

88 Dutch law: Lessing 1983.

88 Picasso snob: Koestler 1964, 103.

89 van Meegeren's argument: Lessing 1983, 60.

90 Knowledge and pleasure: Danto 1981, 14.

90 Sex and forgery: Koestler 1964; see also Lessing 1983.

91 Art as performance: Dutton 1983a, 176; see also Wollheim 1980.

92 Forgery as historically specific: Julius 2002.

92 Famous sweater: Johnson and Jacobs 2001.

93 Speeding up the music: Dutton 1983b.

94 A child can't do it: Yenawine 1991.

94 Aristotle on despised animals and corpses: Danto 1981.

CHAPTER 4: GOOD AND EVIL

101 Whiny war criminals: Baumeister 1997.

101 Capone excuse: Quoted by Stengel 2000, 200.

101 Gacy excuse: Quoted by Baumeister 1997, 50.

101 Augustine on evil: Wills 1999.

102 Gilmore and Bianchi quotes: Hatfield, Cacioppo, and Rapson 1994, 98–99.

102 Bundy excuse: Quoted by Dillard 2000, 21.

103 Psychopaths: Blair 1995; Hare 1993; Hatfield et al. 1994.

103 The genetics of empathy: Zahn-Waxler et al. 1992.

103 Psychopathic monkeys: Harlow and Harlow 1962.

104 Kin selection and morality: Dawkins 1976; Hamilton 1963, 1964; Maynard Smith 1964; see Pinker 1997 for review.

106 **Irony of selfish genes:** Pinker 1997.

106 **Altruism in vampire bats:** Wilkinson 1984.

107 **Good doggy:** Smuts 1999, quoted in Nussbaum 2001, 124.

107 **Debate over altruism:** Cronin 1992.

107 **Darwin on saddles:** Darwin 1964 [1859].

108 **Problems with group selection:** Dawkins 1976; Williams 1966; but see also Sober and Wilson 1998 for a group selection theory that is consistent with the proposal discussed below.

108 **Reciprocal altruism:** Axelrod 1984; Cosmides and Tooby 1992; Dawkins 1976; Hamilton 1963, 1964; Maynard Smith 1964; Trivers, 1971, 1985.

109 **Bad teeth:** Dawkins 1979.

109 **Emotions as adaptations:** Frank 1988; Pinker 1997; Salovey, Mayer, and Caruso 2002; Trivers 1971, 1985.

110 **Emotions and the law:** See Bandes 1999; Nussbaum 1999; Pizarro 2000.

110 **Emotions on *Star Trek*:** Pinker 1997, 372; Hanley 1997.

111 **Men with blunted emotions:** Damasio 1994, quote on 36.

112 **Successful psychopaths?:** Hare 1993.

112 **People born without pain:** Melzack and Wall 1983.

113 **The conventional/moral distinction in psychopaths:** Blair 1995.

113 **Emotions as key to morality:** Nussbaum 2001; Hoffman 2000; Kagan 1994.

114 **Crying babies:** Simmer 1971.

114 **Shocking rats and monkeys:** See Hauser 2000 for review.

114 **Stroke aimed:** Smith 1976 [1759].

114 **Emotional contagion:** Hatfield et al. 1994; see also Gladwell 2000.

115 **Arm-wrestling and stuttering:** Berger and Hadley 1975.

115 **Blindingly fast imitation:** Davis 1985.

115 **Mirror neurons:** Gallese and Goldman 1998.

115 **Bodily motions and emotion:** James 1950 [1890], 326.

116 **Pens in the mouth:** Strack, Martin, and Stepper 1988.

116 **Nodding to headphones:** Wells and Petty 1980.

116 **Muster Salesman:** Gladwell 2000, 73.

117 **Reagan as great communicator:** McHugo et al. 1985.

117 **Philosophical worries about the relationship between empathy and compassion:** See Nussbaum 1999, 2001.

117 **Letter to the Nazis:** Cited in Glover 1999, 379–380.

117 **Aristotle on limits of empathy:** Nussbaum 2001.

118 **Evidence for empathy's link with compassion:** See Hoffman 2000 for review of the extensive experimental literature on this topic.

118 **The importance of others' happiness:** Smith 1976 [1759] 3.

119 **Baby mimics:** Field et al. 1982; Meltzoff and Moore 1977, 1983; Haviland and Lelwica 1987; Termine and Izard 1988.

119 **Sensitive babies:** Martin and Clark 1982; Sagi and Hoffman 1976; Simmer 1971.

119 **Developing responses to others' pain:** Hoffman 2000; see also Eisenberg and Fabes 1991; Harris 1989; Kagan 1984.

119 **Example of an empathetic child:** Hoffman, 1981, 110.

121 **Guilt in one- and two-year-olds:** Zahn-Waxler and Robinson 1995.

121 **The emergence of the moral emotions:** Lewis 2000a, 2000b.

121 **Morality in the first year of life?:** Draghi-Lorenz, Reddy, and Costall 2001; Hay, Nash, and Pederson 1981; Reddy 2000.

122 **Are we moral philosophers?:** De Waal 1996, 209.

CHAPTER 5: THE MORAL CIRCLE

123 **Depraved children:** quoted by Keil 2004.

124 **Disagreement about the beginning of life:** Turiel and Neff 2000, 276.

125 **Knowing more about homosexuality:** Posner 1992.

125 **Slave of the passions:** Hume 1969 [1739], 462.

125 **Intuitions as weapons:** Wright 1994, 328.

125 **Reasoning is post hoc:** Haidt 2001, 814.

125 **Special period for language learning:** Newport 1990.

126 **No best language:** McWhorter 2002.

126 **Special period for morality learning:** Haidt 2001; Harris 1998.

126 **Herodotus on treatment of the dead:** Quoted in Blackburn 2001, 20.

127 **Lawyers, not judges:** Haidt 2001.

127 **Moral dumbfounding:** Haidt, Koller, and Dias 1993.

128 **Taboo thoughts:** Fiske and Tetlock 1997; Tetlock et al. 2000.

129 **The importance of moral deliberation:** Pizarro and Bloom 2002.

130 **Americans on morality:** Wolfe 2001.

131 **The moral majority:** Wolfe 2001, 196–197.

132 **Civil rights struggle:** Coles 1986.

132 **Abortion decision:** Gilligan 1982.

132 **Moral vegetarians:** Amato and Partridge 1989, 36–37.

134 **Enthusiastic participants in genocide:** for instance, Goldhagen 1996; Naimark 2001; Powers 2002.

134 **Prevalence of hunter-gatherer murder:** Pinker 2003.

134 **Biblical command as illustration of moral change:** Singer 1981.

135 **Moral circle:** Singer 1981.

135 **Diffusion of sympathy:** Darwin 1874, 283.

136 **The Wari:** Pinker 1997.

136 **Reminders of death:** Goldenberg et al. 2001.

136 **Killing animals, Hitler, and Stalin:** Quoted in Amato and Partridge 1989, 28.

137 **Rawls on justice and animals:** Rawls 1971, 512.

137 **A special obligation to neighbors and countrymen?:** See Nussbaum and Cohen 2002.

138 **Impartiality in all moral and religious systems:** Singer 1981.

139 **Justifying your action:** Hume 1957 [1751] section IX, part 1, quoted in Singer 1981, 93.

139 **Impartiality and generalization:** Darwin 1874, 285–286; Singer 2000, 267; see also McGinn 1979.

141 **Kennedy's appeal:** Quoted in Frady 2002, 120.

142 **The relationship between reason and morality:** See also Hoffman 2000; Nussbaum 2001; Pizarro 2000; Solomon 1999.

142 **Veil of ignorance:** Rawls 1971.

143 **Empathy and Rawls:** Hoffman 2000.

144 **Controlling the situation you find yourself in:** Elster 2000; Pizarro and Bloom 2002; Schelling 1984.

144 **Grabbing a cookie:** Mischel and Ebbesen 1970.

144 **Appeal from homeless man:** Shaw, Batson, and Todd 1994.

145 **Rational slave owners:** Chomsky 1988; Fredrickson 2002.

145 **Nazi doctors:** Lifton 1986.

145 **Fast-acting Belgians:** Elster 2000.

146 **Not zero-sum:** Wright 2000.

147 **They built my minivan:** Quoted in Pinker 2002, 320.

147 **Familiarity breeds respect:** Allport 1954; Pettigrew 1998; Pettigrew and Tropp 2000.

148 **Seeing humanity in wartime:** Glover 1999, quotes on 53.

149 **Forcing children to take others' perspectives:** Hoffman 1981, 2000.

149 **Greek tragedies:** Nussbaum 2001, 429.

149 **Power of kin metaphors:** Pinker 2002; Solomon 1999.

151 **Moral differences:** Shweder 1994, 26.

152 **Judgments vs. conventions:** Nucci and Turiel 1993; Turiel 1998.

CHAPTER 6: THE BODY AND SOUL EMOTION

155 **Feces as child/feces as penis:** Freud 1962 [1905].

156 **Miller's fastidious children:** Miller 1997.

157 **The Garcia effect:** Garcia, Ervin, and Koelling 1966; Rozin 1986.

158 **Research on disgust:** Rozin and Fallon 1987; Rozin et al. 1997; Rozin, Haidt, and McCauley 2000.

158 **Deadly houseplants:** Cashdan 1994.

159 **Cockroaches, bedpans, and feces-shaped fudge:** Rozin, Millman, and Nemeroff 1986.

159 **Contamination and magic:** Nemeroff and Rozin 2000; Frazer 1959 [1890].

160 **Fooled by television:** Pinker 1997.

161 **The gun game:** Russo 2001, 440.

161 **Disgust as a reaction formation:** Freud 1989 [1930].

162 **Anomaly and disgust:** Douglas 1984.

162 **Problems with Douglas's theory:** See also Miller 1997.

163 **Don't share the disgust:** Leach 1989, 317.

165 **Phobias in people and other primates:** Mineka and Cook 1993.

165 **Disgust needs to be flexible:** Pinker 1997.

166 **Small range of acceptable foods:** Pinker 1997, 380; Darwin 1998 [1872], 257.

166 **Picky children:** Cashdan 1994.

167 **Grasshopper and dog doo:** See Rozin et al. 2000 for review.

167 **Contamination studies with children:** Siegal and Share 1990; Siegal 1995; Siegal and Peterson 1996.

168 **Army recruits:** Peryam 1963.

169 **Whipped cream and hamburger:** Rozin et al. 1986.

169 **Questionnaire studies:** Haidt, McCauley, and Rozin 1994; see also Rozin et al. 2000.

170 **Extending disgust beyond food:** Rozin et al. 2000, 642.

172 **Disgust as metaphor:** Johnson 1993; Pinker 2002.

173 **Disgust as damning:** Miller 1997, 9.

173 **Cloning is disgusting:** Kass 2001, 33; Miller 1998, 86–87.

174 **Controversy about "petophilia":** Singer 2001. The responses to Singer's article are summarized by Saletan 2001, who begins with "Years ago, advocates of sexual abstinence came up with a clever motto to instill chastity in youngsters: 'Pet your dog, not your date,' they preached. They may live to regret those words."

175 **Disgust as a poor moral guide:** Nussbaum 2001; Pinker 2002; though see Kahan 1999 for a measured defense of the moral utility of disgust.

175 **Other people's clothes:** Nemeroff and Rozin 1994.

176 **Disgust as a weapon:** Nussbaum 2001, 347.

176 **Voltaire on the Jews, the Jews on the Host:** Miller 1997.

176 **Causes of genocide:** See Glover 1999; Naimark 2001; Sternberg 2001.

177 **Treatment of Jews/Armenians:** Nussbaum 2001, 347; Naimark 2001.

177 **Primo Levi on the acts of the Nazis:** Levi 1988, 70–71, quoted in Nussbaum 2001, 348.

178 **Surviving the concentration camps:** Des Pres 1976.

178 **Diminishing people:** Glover 1999, 37.

178 **Pirate torture:** Wills 1999.

179 **Overriding disgust:** Fry 1992, 84.

179 **The mystery of the toothbrush:** Freud 1962 [1905].

180 **Signal of a failing marriage:** Gottman 1995.

180 **Attitude during autopsy:** Gawande 2001.

181 **Reassuring rituals:** Nemeroff and Rozin 1992; also Kass 1994.

181 **Sixteenth-century manners:** Quoted in Elias 1982, 119. See also Kass 1994; Miller 1997.

182 **Initiation rites:** Miller 1997.

182 **Do you want to see something disgusting?:** Haidt 2003.

182 **A popular book on the brain:** Greenfield 2000, 159.

183 **A shift in perspective:** Koestler 1964.

183 **The cruel nature of laughter:** Provine 2000; quote from Glover 1999, 49.

184 **Defining humor:** Barry 1991, 7.

184 **Functions of laughter:** Pinker 1997.

185 **Mechanical encrusted on the living:** Bergson 1911.

185 **Slapstick:** Dale 2000, 14.

CHAPTER 7: THEREFORE I AM

189 The problem of reanimation: Taylor 2002.

190 Double funerals: Boyer 2001; Taylor 2002.

190 American religious views: Gallup and Newport 1991; Shermer 2000.

192 Conjoined twins: Campbell 2003.

192 Man with little brain: Lewin 1980; **as evidence for a nonmaterialist position:** Dembski 1999.

193 Phantom limbs: Ramachandran and Blakeslee 1998; Sachs 1985.

193 Descartes' skepticism: Descartes 1968 [1641]·

194 Cogito ergo sum: Flanagan 2002, 174, notes that Augustine was there first when he wrote "*Si fallor sum*" ("If I doubt, I am"). For problems with Descartes' argument, see, for example, Flanagan 1984.

196 Soulless clones: Doniger 1998.

197 Ensoulment and its problems: Pinker 2002.

198 Piaget on indiscriminate children: Piaget 1929, 55.

199 Young children are dualists: Wellman 1990, 50.

199 Mental entities vs. physical entities: Estes, Wellman, and Woolley 1989; Wellman and Estes 1986.

199 What children think the brain does: Gottfried, Gelman, and Schultz 1999; Johnson 1990, 2000; Johnson and Wellman 1982; Lillard 1996.

200 People can get along without thinking: Flavell, Green, and Flavell 1995, 1998.

201 Transfer of kindness: Johnson 1990.

201 Change of heart: Sylvia and Novak 1997, 165; see also Gelman 2003.

201 Troubles with the pilot metaphor: Flanagan 1984.

202 Brionny's experience of the will: McEwan 2002, 35–36; see also Wegner 2002 for a review of research on the experience of willful action.

203 Augustine on bodies and souls: Wills 1999, 133.

204 Downloading your mind: Kurzweil 1999.

204 Resurrection of Christ: Pagels 1979.

204 Proper treatment of the dead: Lithwick 2002.

205 Naughty people: Sully 1896, cited by Harris 2000, 171–172.

205 Confusion about death: Carey 1985, 27.

206 A full understanding of death: Lazar and Torney-Purta 1991; Lutz 2003; Slaughter, Jaakkola, and Carey 1999.

206 Burial artifacts: White 1993.

207 Children believe that the mind outlives the body: Bering and Bjork-lund, under review.

CHAPTER 8: GODS, SOULS, AND SCIENCE

209 Lateran proclamation on God and the duality of humans: Quoted in Flanagan 2002.

209 Living forests and other deities: Boyer 2001.

210 **Compromise theory of supernatural beings:** Boyer 2001, see also Sperber 1996.

211 **Supernatural templates:** Boyer 2001, 78–79.

212 **What sort of things people will remember:** see Barrett 2000 for review.

213 **The astonishing hypothesis:** Crick 1994.

214 **Theological correctness:** Barrett and Keil 1996; see also Barrett 2000.

214 **Catholics on heaven and hell:** Flanagan 2002.

214 **Anthromorphic perspectives on God:** Bowker 2002.

215 **Mean stupid spirits:** Boyer 2001.

215 **Yahweh as insecure:** Stengel 2000, 68.

215 **Anthromorphic deity:** Barrett 1998; Barrett and Keil 1996; Barrett and VanOrman 1996.

217 **Magic box and magic water:** Subbotsky 1993.

217 **Monster box:** Harris et al. 1991.

218 **Children do not believe in magic after all:** See also Taylor 1999; Woolley 2000.

218 **Pencil in the box:** Woolley and Phelps 1994.

218 **Make-believe vs. real-life:** Harris et al. 1991.

218 **Cyanide:** Rozin et al. 1990.

218 **Horror movies, Marcus Welby, and Little Nell:** Taylor 1999.

219 **Imaginary companions:** Taylor 1999; see also Singer and Singer 1990.

220 **Wishing and praying:** Woolley 2000.

220 **Santa Claus and God:** Clark 1995; Taylor 1999.

221 **God as human:** Goldman 1964.

221 **God vs. the child's best friend:** Giménez and Harris 2000; see also Barrett, Richert, and Driesenga 2001.

221 **God's limited powers:** *New York Times,* A10, 18 July 2002.

221 **Happy tulips:** Coley 1995.

221 **Autistic views of God:** Grandin 1995, 191 and 200; Schneider 1999, 54, both cited in Bering 2002, 14.

222 **Language organ:** Chomsky 1980; Pinker 1994.

223 **Square peg and round hole:** Putnam 1975b.

224 **Science and religion are separate:** Gould 1999.

225 **Empirical claims by religions:** Crews 2001; Flanagan 2002; Sterelny 2001.

225 **Clash between religion and cognitive science:** Cited in Pinker 2002, 186–187.

226 **Retaining the beautiful, true, and inspiring:** Flanagan 2002, xvi.

226 **Fulfilled atheist:** Dawkins 1986.

REFERENCES

Ackerman, J. 2001. *Chance in the House of Fate: A Natural History of Heredity.* New York: Houghton Mifflin.

Ahn, W.-K. 2002. "Conceptual and Causal Knowledge." Paper presented at Yale University, Department of Psychology, November 11.

Allport, G. W. 1954. *The Nature of Prejudice.* Reading, Mass.: Addison-Wesley.

Almquist, A. J., and J. E. Cronin. 1988. "Fact, Fancy and Myth on Human Evolution." *Current Anthropology:* 29, 520–522.

Alvarez, A. 2001. *Poker: Bets, Bluffs, and Bad Beats.* San Francisco: Chronicle Books.

Amato, R., and S. A. Partridge. 1989. *The New Vegetarians: Promoting Health and Protecting Life.* New York: Plenum Press.

Atran, S. 1998. "Folk Biology and the Anthropology of Science: Cognitive Universals and Cultural Particulars." *Behavioral and Brain Sciences* 21: 547–609.

Axelrod, R. 1984. *The Evolution of Cooperation.* New York: Basic Books.

Baillargeon, R. 2002. "The Acquisition of Physical Knowledge in Infancy: A Summary in Eight Lessons." In U. Goswami, ed., *Blackwell Handbook of Childhood Cognitive Development.* Cambridge, Mass.: Blackwell.

Baillargeon, R., E. S. Spelke, and S. Wasserman. 1985. "Object Permanence in Five-Month-Old Infants." *Cognition* 20: 191–208.

Baldwin, D. A., E. M. Markman, and R. L. Melartin. 1993. "Infants' Ability to Draw Inferences About Nonobvious Object Properties: Evidence from Exploratory Play." *Cognitive Development* 64: 711–728.

Bandes, S. A., ed. 1999. *The Passions of Law.* New York: New York University Press.

Baron-Cohen, S. 1995. *Mindblindness: An Essay on Autism and Theory of Mind.* Cambridge, Mass.: MIT Press.

———. 2002. "The Extreme Male Brain Theory of Autism." *Trends in Cognitive Sciences* 6: 248–254.

Baron-Cohen, S., A. M. Leslie, and U. Frith, 1985. "Does the Autistic Child Have a 'Theory of Mind'?" *Cognition* 21: 37–46.

Barrett, J. L. 1998. "Cognitive Constraints on Hindu Concepts of the Divine." *Journal for the Scientific Study of Religion* 37: 608–619.

———. 2000. "Exploring the Natural Foundations of Religion." *Trends in Cognitive Sciences* 4: 29–34.

Barrett, J. L., and F. C. Keil. 1996. "Conceptualizing a Non-natural Entity: Anthropomorphism in God Concepts." *Cognitive Psychology* 31: 219–247.

Barrett, J. L., R. A. Richert, and A. Driesenga. 2001. "God's Beliefs Versus Mother's: The Development of Nonhuman Agent Concepts." *Child Development* 72: 50–65.

Barrett, J. L., and B. VanOrman. 1996. "The Effects of Image Use in Worship on God Concepts." *Journal of Psychology and Christianity* 15: 38–45.

Barry, D. 1991. *Dave Barry Talks Back*. New York: Crown Publishers.

Bartsch, K., and H. M. Wellman. 1995. *Children Talk About the Mind*. New York: Oxford University Press.

Basalla, G. 1988. *The Evolution of Technology*. Cambridge: Cambridge University Press.

Baumeister, R. G. 1997. *Evil: Inside Human Violence and Cruelty*. New York: Freeman.

Beilin, H., and E. G. Pearlman. 1991. "Children's Iconic Realism: Object vs. Property Realism." In H. W. Reese, ed., *Advances in Child Development and Behavior,* vol. 23. New York: Academic Press.

Berger, S. M., and S. W. Hadley. 1975. "Some Effects of a Model's Performance on an Observer's Electromyographic Activity." *American Journal of Psychology* 88: 263–276.

Bergson, H. 1911. *Laughter: An Essay on the Meaning of the Comic.* London: Macmillan.

Bering, J. M. 2002. "The Existential Theory of Mind." *Review of General Psychology* 6: 3–24.

Bering, J. M., and D. F. Bjorklund. Under review. "Simulation Constraints and the Natural Emergence of Afterlife Reasoning as a Developmental Regularity."

Bertenthal, B. I., D. R. Proffitt, N. B. Spetner, and M. A. Thomas, 1985. "The Development of Infant Sensitivity to Biomechanical Motions." *Child Development* 56: 531–543.

Birch, S. A. J., and P. Bloom. 2003. "Children Are Cursed: An Asymmetric Bias in Mentalistic Attribution." *Psychological Science* 14: 283–286.

———. Under review. "The Curse of Knowledge in Reasoning About False Beliefs."

Blackburn, S. 2001. *Being Good: A Short Introduction to Ethics*. New York: Oxford University Press.

Blair, J. R. 1995. "A Cognitive Developmental Approach to Morality: Investigating the Psychopath." *Cognition* 57: 1–29.

Bloom, P. 1994. "Generativity Within Language and Other Cognitive Domains." *Cognition* 51: 177–189.

———. 1996. "Intention, History, and Artifact Concepts." *Cognition* 60: 1–29.

———. 1998. "Theories of Artifact Categorization." *Cognition* 66: 87–93.

———. 2000. *How Children Learn the Meanings of Words*. Cambridge, Mass.: MIT Press.

Bloom, P., F. Abell, F. Happé, and U. Frith. Under review. "Picture Naming in Children with Autism."

Bloom, P., and T. German. 2000. "Two Reasons to Abandon the False Belief Task as a Test of Theory of Mind." *Cognition* 77: B25-B32.

Bloom, P., and F. C. Keil. 2001. "Thinking Through Language." *Mind and Language* 16: 351–367.

Bloom, P., and L. Markson. 1997. "Children's Naming of Representations." Poster presented to the Society for Research in Child Development, April 4–6.

——. 1998. "Intention and Analogy in Children's Naming of Pictorial Representations." *Psychological Science* 9: 200–204.

Bloom, P., and C. Veres. 1999. "The Perceived Intentionality of Groups." *Cognition* 71: B1-B9.

Borges, J. L. 1964. "Funes the Memorious." In *Labyrinths: Selected Stories and Other Writings*. New York: New Directions.

Bowker, G. C., and S. L. Star. 1999. *Sorting Things Out: Classification and Its Consequences*. Cambridge, Mass.: MIT Press.

Bowker, J. 2002. *God: A Brief History*. New York: DK Publishing.

Bretherton, I. 1992. "Social Referencing, Intentional Communication, and the Interfacing of Minds in Infancy." In D. Frye and C. Moore, eds., *Children's Theories of Mind: Mental States and Social Understanding*. New York: Plenum Press.

Boyer, P. 2001. *Religion Explained*. New York: Basic Books.

Brown, D. E. 1991. *Human Universals*. New York: McGraw Hill.

Bryson, B. 1992. *Neither Here Nor There: Travels in Europe*. New York: Avon.

Call, J., and M. Tomasello. 1994. "The Production and Comprehension of Referential Pointing By Orangutans *Pongo pygmaeus*." *Journal of Comparative Psychology* 108: 307–317.

Campbell, A. 2003. "Contestable Bodies: Law, Medicine, and the Case of Conjoined Twins." Unpublished manuscript, Carleton University (Ottawa).

Campos, J. J., and C. R. Stenberg. 1981. "Perception, Appraisal, and Emotion: The Onset of Social Referencing." In M. E. Lamb and L. R. Sherrod, eds., *Infant Social Cognition: Empirical and Theoretical Considerations*. Hillsdale, N.J.: Erlbaum.

Carey, S. 1985. *Conceptual Change in Childhood*. Cambridge, Mass.: MIT Press.

——. 2004. "The Origin of Concepts." Unpublished manuscript. Department of Psychology, Harvard University.

Carruthers, P. 1996. *Language, Thought, and Consciousness*. Cambridge: Cambridge University Press.

Cashdan, E. 1994. "A Sensitive Period for Learning About Food." *Human Nature* 5: 279–291.

——. 1998. "Adaptiveness of Food Learning and Food Aversions in Children." *Social Science Information* 37: 613–632.

Charman, T., J. Swettenham, S. Baron-Cohen, A. Cox, G. Baird, and A. Drew. 1997. "Infants with Autism: An Investigation of Empathy, Pretend Play, Joint Attention, and Imitation." *Developmental Psychology* 33: 781–789.

Chomsky, N. 1980. *Rules and Representations*. New York: Columbia University Press.

——. 1988. *Language and Problems of Knowledge: The Managua Lectures*. Cambridge, Mass.: MIT Press.

Clark, C. D. 1995. *Flights of Fancy, Leaps of Faith: Children's Myth in Contemporary America*. Chicago: University of Chicago Press.

Coles, R. 1986. *The Moral Life of Children: How Children Struggle with Questions of Moral Choice in the United States and Elsewhere.* Boston: Houghton Mifflin.

Coley, J. D. 1995. "Emerging Differentiation of Folkbiology and Folkpsychology: Attributions of Biological and Psychological Properties to Living Things." *Child Development* 66, 1856–1874.

Corkum, V., and C. Moore. 1995. "Development of Joint Visual Attention in Infants." In C. Moore and P. Dunham, eds., *Joint Attention: Its Origin and Role in Development.* Hillsdale, N.J.: Erlbaum.

Cosmides, L., and J. Tooby. 1992. "Cognitive Adaptations for Social Exchange." In J. H. Barkow, L. Cosmides, and J. Tooby, eds., *The Adapted Mind: Evolutionary Psychology and the Generation of Culture.* New York: Oxford University Press.

Cosmides, L., J. Tooby, and R. Kurzban. 2003. "Perceptions of Race." *Trends in Cognitive Sciences* 7: 173–179.

Cox, M. 1992. *Children's Drawings.* London: Penguin Books.

Crews, F. 2001. "Saving Us from Darwin." *New York Review of Books*, Oct. 4.

Crick, F. 1994. *The Astonishing Hypothesis: The Scientific Search for the Soul.* New York: Simon & Schuster.

Cronin, H. 1992. *The Ant and the Peacock.* New York: Cambridge University Press.

Dale, A. 2000. *Comedy Is a Man in Trouble.* Minneapolis, Minn.: University of Minnesota Press.

D'Andrade, R. 1987. "A Folk Model of the Mind." In D. Holland and N. Quinn, eds., *Cultural Models in Language and Thought.* Cambridge: Cambridge University Press.

Damasio, A. R. 1994. *Descartes' Error: Emotion, Reason, and the Human Brain.* New York: Putnam.

Danto, A. 1964. "The Artworld." *Journal of Philosophy* 61: 571–584.

———. 1981. *The Transfiguration of the Commonplace.* Cambridge, Mass.: Harvard University Press.

———. 1986. "The Philosophical Disenfranchisement of Art." In A. Danto, ed., *The Philosophical Disenfranchisement of Art.* New York: Columbia University Press.

Darwin, C. R. 1874. *The Descent of Man, and Selection in Relation in Sex.* 2nd edition. New York: Hurst.

———. 1964 [1859]. *On the Origin of Species.* Cambridge, Mass.: MIT Press.

———. 1998 [1872]. *The Expression of the Emotions in Man and Animals.* Oxford: Oxford University Press.

Davies, S. 1991. *Definitions of Art.* Ithaca, N.Y.: Cornell University Press.

Davis, M. R. 1985. "Perceptual and Affective Reverberation Components." In A. B. Goldstein and G. Y. Michaels, eds., *Empathy: Development, Training, and Consequences.* Hillsdale, N.J.: Erlbaum.

Dawkins, R. 1976. *The Selfish Gene.* New York: Oxford University Press.

———. 1979. "Twelve Misunderstandings of Kin Selection." *Zeitschrift für Tierpsychologie* 51: 331–367.

―――. 1986. *The Blind Watchmaker: Why the Evidence of Evolution Reveals a Universe Without Design.* New York: Norton.

Dawson, G., A. N. Meltzoff, J. Osterling, J. Rinaldi, and E. Brown. 1998. "Children with Autism Fail to Orient to Naturally Occurring Social Stimuli." *Journal of Autism and Developmental Disorders* 28: 479–485.

DeLoache, J. S. 1995. "Early Understanding and Use of Symbols: The Model Model." *Current Directions in Psychological Science* 4: 109–113.

DeLoache, J. S., and N. M. Burns. 1994. "Early Understanding of the Representational Function of Pictures." *Cognition* 52: 83–110.

DeLoache, J. S., and D. Marzolf. 1995. "The Use of Dolls to Interview Young Children: Issues of Symbolic Representation." *Journal of Experimental Child Psychology* 60: 155–173.

DeLoache, J. S., K. F. Miller, and K. S. Rosengren. 1997. "The Credible Shrinking Room: Very Young Children's Performance with Symbolic and Nonsymbolic Relations." *Psychological Science* 8: 308–313.

DeLoache, J. S., S. L. Pierroutsakos, D. H. Uttal, K. S. Rosengren, and A. Gottlieb. 1998. "Grasping the Nature of Pictures." *Psychological Science* 9: 205–210.

DeLoache, J. S., M. Strauss, and J. Maynard. 1979. "Picture Perception in Infancy." *Infant Behavior and Development* 2: 77–89.

Dembski, W. A. 1999. "Are We Spiritual Machines?" *First Things* 96: 25–31.

Dennett, D. C. 1978. "Response to Premack and Woodruff: Does the Chimpanzee Have a Theory of Mind?" *Behavioral and Brain Sciences* 4: 568–570.

―――. 1990. "The Interpretation of Texts, People, and Other Artifacts." *Philosophy and Phenomenological Research* 50: 177–194.

―――. 1994. "Get Real." *Philosophical Topics* 22: 505–568.

―――. 1995. *Darwin's Dangerous Idea: Evolution and the Meanings of Life.* New York: Simon & Schuster.

―――. 1996. *Kinds of Minds.* New York: Basic Books.

Des Pres, T. 1976. *The Survivor.* New York: Oxford University Press.

Descartes, R. 1968 [1641]. Meditations. In E. Haldane and G. Ross, ed., *The Philosophical Works of Descartes.* 2 vols. Cambridge: Cambridge University Press.

Diamond, A. 1991. "Neuropsychological Insights into the Meaning of Object Concept Development." In S. Carey and R. Gelman, eds., *The Epigenesis of Mind: Essays on Biology and Cognition.* Hillsdale, N.J.: Erlbaum.

Dickie, G. 1984. *The Art Circle.* New York: Haven Publications.

Diesendruck, G. 2001. "Essentialism in Brazilian Children's Extensions of Animal Names." *Developmental Psychology* 37: 49–60.

Diesendruck, G., S. A. Gelman, and K. Lebowitz. 1998. "Conceptual and Linguistic Biases in Children's Word Learning." *Developmental Psychology* 34: 823–839.

Diesendruck, G., L. Markson, and P. Bloom. 2003. "Children's Reliance on Creator's Intent in Extending Names for Artifacts." *Psychological Science* 14: 164–168.

Dillard, A. 2000. *For the Time Being.* New York: Vintage Books.

Dissanayake, E. 1992. *Homo Aestheticus: Where Art Comes from and Why.* New York: Free Press.

Doniger, W. 1998. "Sex and the Mythological Clone." In M. C. Nussbaum and C. R. Sunstein, eds., *Clones and Clones: Facts and Fantasies About Human Cloning*. New York: Norton.

Douglas, M. 1984. *Purity and Danger: An Analysis of Concepts of Pollution and Taboo*. New York: Routledge.

Draghi-Lorenz, R., V. Reddy, and A. Costall. 2001. "Rethinking the Development of 'Nonbasic' Emotions: A Critical Review of Existing Theories." *Developmental Review* 21: 263–304.

Dupré, J. 1993. *The Disorder of Things: Metaphysical Foundations of the Disunity of Science*. Cambridge, Mass.: Harvard University Press.

Dutton, D. 1983a. "Artistic Crimes." In *The Forger's Art: Forgery and the Philosophy of Art*. Berkeley and Los Angeles: University of California Press.

———. 1983b. Preface. *The Forger's Art: Forgery and the Philosophy of Art*. Berkeley and Los Angeles: University of California Press.

Eisenberg, N., and R. A. Fabes. 1991. "Prosocial Behavior and Empathy: A Multimethod Developmental Perspective." In M. S. Clark, ed., *Prosocial Behavior*. Newbury Park, Calif.: Sage Publications.

Ekman, P., and Friesen, W. V. 1975. *Unmasking the Face*. Englewood Cliffs, N.J.: Prentice-Hall.

Elias, N. 1982. *The History of Manners*. New York: Random House.

Elkins, J. 2001. *Pictures and Tears: A History of People Who Have Cried in Front of Paintings*. New York: Routledge.

Elster, J. 2000. *Ulysses Unbound: Studies in Rationality, Precommitment, and Constraints*. New York: Cambridge University Press.

Estes, D., H. M. Wellman, and J. D. Woolley. 1989. "Children's Understanding of Mental Phenomena." In H. Reese, ed., *Advances in Child Development and Behavior*. New York: Academic Press.

Evans, E. M. 1997. "Beyond Scopes: Why Creationism Is Here to Stay." In K. S. Rosengren, C. N. Johnson, and L. Harris, eds., *Imagining the Impossible: Magical, Scientific, and Religious Thinking in Children*. New York: Cambridge University Press.

———. 2001. "Cognitive and Contextual Factors in the Emergence of Diverse Belief Systems: Creation Versus Evolution." *Cognitive Psychology* 42: 217–266.

Evans, M. E., S. A. Gelman, J. M. Vidic, and D. Poling. 1996. "Artificialism Revisited: Preschoolers' Explanations for the Origins of Artifacts and Natural Kinds." Paper presented at the Conference on Human Development, Birmingham, Alabama, March 29–31.

Evans, M. E., S. F. Stewart, and D. A. Poling. 1997. "Humans Have a Privileged Status: Parental Explanations for the Origins of Human and Non-human Species." Paper presented at the Biennial Meeting of the Society for Research in Child Development, Washington, D.C., April 3–6.

Field, T. M., D. Cohen, R. Garcia, and R. Greenberg. 1984. "Mother-Stranger Face Discrimination by the Newborn." *Infant Behavior and Development* 7: 19–25.

Field, T. M., N. Vega-Lahr, F. Scafidi, and S. Goldstein. 1986. "Effects of Material Unreliability on Mother-Infant Interactions." *Infant Behavior and Development* 9: 473–478.

Field, T. M., R. Woodson, R. Greenberg, and D. Cohen. 1982. "Discrimination and Imitation of Facial Expressions by Neonates." *Science* 218: 179-181.

Fiske, A., and E. Tetlock. 1997. "Taboo Trade-offs: Reactions to Transactions That Transgress the Spheres of Justice." *Political Psychology* 18: 255–297.

Flanagan, O. 1984. *The Science of the Mind.* Cambridge, Mass.: MIT Press.

———. 2002. *The Problem of the Soul: Two Visions of Mind and How to Reconcile Them.* New York: Basic Books.

Flavell, J. H., F. L. Green, and E. R. Flavell. 1995. "Young Children's Knowledge About Thinking." *Monographs of the Society for Research in Child Development* 60, no. 1, serial no. 243.

———. 1998. "The Mind Has a Mind of Its Own: Developing Knowledge of Mental Uncontrollability." *Cognitive Development* 13: 127–138.

Fodor, J. A. 1992. "A Theory of the Child's Theory of Mind." *Cognition* 44: 283–296.

———. 1993. "*Déjà Vu* All Over Again: How Danto's Aesthetics Recapitulates the Philosophy of Mind." In M. Rollins, ed., *Danto and His Critics.* Cambridge, Mass.: Blackwell.

Fox, R., and C. McDaniel, 1982. "The Perception of Biological Motion by Human Infants." *Science* 218: 486–487.

Frady, M. 2002. *Martin Luther King, Jr.* New York: Penguin.

Frank, R. H. 1988. *Passions Within Reason: The Strategic Role of the Emotions.* New York: Norton.

Frazer, J. G. 1959 [1890]. *The Golden Bough: A Study in Magic and Religion.* London: Macmillan.

Fredrickson, G. M. 2002. *Racism: A Short Introduction.* Princeton, N.J.: Princeton University Press.

Freeman, N. H. 1991. "The Theory of Art That Underpins Children's Naïve Realism." *Visual Arts Research* 17: 65–75.

Freud, S. 1962 [1905]. *Three Essays on the Theory of Sexuality.* New York: Basic Books.

———. 1989 [1930]. *Civilization and Its Discontents.* New York: Norton.

Friedman, W. 1990. *About Time: Inventing the Fourth Dimension.* Cambridge, Mass.: MIT Press.

Fry, S. 1992. *Paperweight.* London: Random House.

Gallese, V., and A. Goldman. 1998. "Mirror Neurons and the Simulation Theory of Mind-Reading." *Trends in Cognitive Sciences* 2: 493–501.

Gallup, G. H., and F. Newport. 1991. "Belief in Paranormal Phenomena Among Adult Americans." *Skeptical Inquirer* 15: 137–146.

Garcia, J., F. R. Ervin, and R. A. Koelling. 1966. "Learning with Prolonged Delay of Reinforcement." *Psychonomic Science* 5: 121–122.

Gardner, H. 1980. *Artful Scribbles: The Significance of Children's Drawings.* London: Jill Norman.

Gaukroger, S. 1995. *Descartes: An Intellectual Biography*. Clarendon: Oxford.

Gawande, A. 2001. "Final Cut: Why Have Doctors Stopped Doing Autopsies?" *The New Yorker*, March 19, 94–99.

Geertz, C. 1983. "'From the Native's Point of View': On the Nature of Anthropological Understanding." In *Local Knowledge: Further Essays in Interpretive Anthropology*. New York: Basic Books.

Gelman, S. A. 2003. *The Essential Child*. New York: Oxford University Press.

Gelman, S. A., and P. Bloom. 2000. "Young Children Are Sensitive to How an Object Was Created When Deciding What to Name It." *Cognition* 76: 91–103.

Gelman, S. A., and K. S. Ebeling. 1998. "Shape and Representational Status in Children's Early Naming." *Cognition* 66: 835–847.

Gelman, S. A., and L. A. Hirschfeld. 1999. "How Biological Is Essentialism?" In S. Atran and D. Medin, eds., *Folkbiology*. Cambridge, Mass.: MIT Press.

Gelman, S. A., and K. E. Kremer. 1991. "Understanding Natural Causes: Children's Explanations of How Objects and Their Properties Originate." *Child Development* 62: 396–414.

Gelman, S. A., and E. M. Markman. 1986. "Categories and Induction in Young Children." *Cognition* 23: 183–209.

———. 1987. "Young Children's Inductions from Natural Kinds: The Role of Categories and Appearances." *Child Development* 58: 1532–1541.

Gelman, S. A., and H. M. Wellman. 1991. "Insides and Essences: Early Understandings of the Nonobvious." *Cognition* 38: 213–244.

Gergely, G., Z. Nádasdy, G. Csibra, and S. Biró. 1995. "Taking the Intentional Stance at 12 Months of Age." *Cognition* 56: 165–193.

Gilligan, C. 1982. *In a Different Voice: Psychological Theory and Women's Development*. Cambridge, Mass.: Harvard University Press.

Giménez, M., and L. Harris. 2000. "Understanding the Impossible: Intimations of Immortality and Omniscience in Early Childhood." Unpublished manuscript. Department of Experimental Psychology, Oxford University.

Gladwell, M. 2000. *The Tipping Point: How Little Things Can Make a Big Difference*. New York: Little, Brown.

Glover, J. 1999. *Humanity: A Moral History of the Twentieth Century*. New Haven: Yale University Press.

Goldenberg, J. L, T. Pyszczynski,, J. Greenberg, S. Solomon, B. Kluck, and R. Cornwell. 2001. "I Am Not an Animal: Morality Salience, Disgust, and the Denial of Human Creatureliness." *Journal of Experimental Psychology: General* 3: 427–435.

Goldhagen, D. J. 1996. *Hitler's Willing Executioners: Ordinary Germans and the Holocaust*. New York: Knopf.

Goldman, R. 1964. *Religious Thinking from Childhood to Adolescence*. London: Routledge & Kegan Paul.

Golomb, C. 1993. "Art and the Young Child: Another Look at the Developmental Question." *Visual Arts Research* 19: 1–15.

Gopnik, A. 1993a. "How We Know Our Minds: The Illusion of First-Person Knowledge of Intentionality." *Behavioral and Brain Sciences* 16: 1–14.

————. 1993b. "Mindblindness." Unpublished manuscript. Department of Psychology, University of California, Berkeley.

Gopnik, A., and A. N. Meltzoff. 1997. *Words, Thoughts, and Theories.* Cambridge, Mass.: MIT Press.

Gopnik, A., A. N. Meltzoff, and P. Kuhl. 1999. *The Scientist in the Crib: What Early Learning Tells Us About the Mind.* New York: William Morrow.

Gottfried, G. M., S. A. Gelman, and H. Schultz. 1999. "Children's Early Understanding of the Brain: From Early Essentialism to Naïve Theory." *Cognitive Development* 14: 147–174.

Gottman, J. 1995. *Why Marriages Succeed or Fail and How You Can Make Yours Last.* New York: Simon & Schuster.

Gould, S. J. 1999. *Rock of Ages: Science and Religion in the Fullness of Life.* New York: Ballantine.

Gould, S. J., and R. C. Lewontin. 1979. "The Spandrels of San Marco and the Panglossian Program: A Critique of the Adaptationist Programme." *Proceedings of the Royal Society of London* 205: 281–288.

Gould, S. J., and E. Vrba. 1982. "Exaptation—A missing term in the Science of Form." *Paleobiology* 8: 4–15.

Grandin, T. 1995. *Thinking in Pictures and Other Reports from My Life with Autism.* New York: Doubleday.

Greenfield, S. 2000. *Brain Power: Working Out the Human Mind.* New York: Houghton Mifflin.

Gutheil, G., P. Bloom, N. Valderrama, and R. Freedman. In press. "The Role of Historical Intuitions in Children's and Adults' Naming of Artifacts." *Cognition.*

Guthrie, S. 1993. *Faces in the Clouds.* New York: Oxford University Press.

Haidt, J. 2001. "The Emotional Dog and Its Rational Tail: A Social Intuitionist Approach to Moral Judgment." *Psychological Review* 108: 814–834.

————. 2003. "The Moral Emotions." In R. J. Davidson, K. R. Scherer, and H. H. Goldsmith, eds., *Handbook of Affective Sciences.* New York: Oxford University Press.

Haidt, J., S. H. Koller, and M. G. Dias. 1993. "Affect, Culture, and Morality, or Is It Wrong to Eat Your Dog?" *Journal of Personality and Social Psychology* 65: 613–628.

Haidt, J., C. McCauley, and P. Rozin, 1994. "Individual Differences in Sensitivity to Disgust: A Scale Sampling Seven Domains of Disgust Elicitors." *Personality and Individual Differences* 16: 701–713.

Hamilton, W. D. 1963. "The Evolution of Altruistic Behavior." *American Naturalist* 97: 354–356.

————. 1964. "The Genetical Evolution of Social Behavior I and II." *Journal of Theoretical Biology* 7: 1–16, 17–52.

Hanley, R. 1997. *The Metaphysics of Star Trek.* New York: Basic Books.

Happé, F. 1996. *Autism: An Introduction to Psychological Theory.* Cambridge, Mass.: Harvard University Press.

Hare, B., M. Brown, C. Williamson, and M. Tomasello. 2002. "The Domestication of Social Cognition in Dogs." *Science* 298: 1634–1636.

Hare, R. D. 1993. *Without Conscience: The Disturbing World of the Psychopaths Around Us.* New York: Guilford Press.

Harlow, H. F., and M. K. Harlow. 1962. "Social Deprivation in Monkeys." *Scientific American* 207: 136–146.

Harris, J. R. 1998. *The Nurture Assumption: Why Children Turn Out the Way They Do.* New York: Free Press.

Harris, P. L. 1989. *Children and Emotion: The Development of Psychological Understanding.* Cambridge, Mass.: Blackwell.

Harris, P. L. 2000. "On Not Falling Down to Earth: Children's Metaphysical Questions." In K. S. Rosengren, C. N. Johnson, and L. Harris, eds., *Imagining the Impossible: Magical, Scientific, and Religious Thinking in Children.* New York: Cambridge University Press.

Harris, P. L., E. Brown, C. Marriott, S. Whittall, and S. Harmer. 1991. "Monsters, Ghosts, and Witches: Testing the Limits of the Fantasy-Reality Distinction in Young Children." *British Journal of Developmental Psychology* 9: 105–123.

Hatfield, E., J. T. Cacioppo, and R. L. Rapson. 1994. *Emotional Contagion.* New York: Cambridge University Press.

Haugeland, J. 1993. "Pattern and Being." In M. Rollins, ed., *Danto and His Critics.* Cambridge, Mass.: Blackwell.

Hauser, M. D. 2000. *Wild Minds: What Animals Really Think.* New York: Henry Holt.

Hauser, M. D., P. MacNeilage, and M. Ware. 1996. "Numerical Representations in Primates: Perceptual or Arithmetic?" *Proceedings of the National Academy of Sciences, USA* 93: 1514–1517.

Haviland, J. M., and M. Lelwica. 1987. "The Induced Affect Response: 10-Week-Old Infants' Responses to Three Emotion Expressions." *Developmental Psychology* 23: 97–104.

Hay, D. F., A. Nash, and J. Pedersen. 1981. "Responses of Six-Month-Olds to the Distress of Their Peers." *Child Development* 52: 1071–1075.

Heath, S. B. 1986. "What No Bedtime Story Means: Narrative Skills at Home and School." In B. S. Schieffelin and E. Ochs, eds., *Language Socialization Across Cultures.* Cambridge: Cambridge University Press.

Heider, F., and M. Simmel. 1944. "An Experimental Study of Apparent Behavior." *American Journal of Psychology* 57: 243–259.

Hirschfeld, L. A. 1996. *Race in the Making.* Cambridge, Mass.: MIT Press.

Hobson, R. P. 2002. *The Cradle of Thought: Exploring the Origins of Thinking.* London: Macmillan.

Hochberg, J., and V. Brooks. 1962. "Pictorial Recognition as an Unlearned Ability: A Study of One Child's Performance." *American Journal of Psychology* 75: 624–628.

Hoffman, M. L. 1981. "Interaction of Affect and Cognition in Empathy." In C. Izard, S. Kagan, and R. Zajonc, eds., *Emotions, Cognition, and Behavior.* New York: Cambridge University Press.

———. 2000. *Empathy and Moral Development: Implications for Caring and Justice.* New York: Cambridge University Press.

Hornby, N. 2000. Introduction. *Speaking with the Angel.* New York: Penguin.

Hubbell, S. 2001. *Shrinking the Cat: Genetic Engineering Before We Knew About Genes.* New York: Houghton Mifflin.

Hull, D. L. 1965. "The Effect of Essentialism on Taxonomy—Two Thousand Years of Stasis." *British Journal for the Philosophy of Science* 15: 314–326.

Hume, D. 1969 [1739]. *A Treatise on Human Nature.* London: Penguin.

———. 1957 [1751]. *An Enquiry Concerning the Principles of Morals.* New York: Liberal Arts Press.

Humphrey, N. 1996. *Leaps of Faith: Science, Miracles, and the Search for Supernatural Consolation.* New York: Springer-Verlag.

Ittelson, W. H. 1996. "Visual Perception of Markings." *Psychonomic Bulletin and Review* 3: 171–187.

James, W. 1950 [1890]. *The Principles of Psychology.* New York: Dover.

Jayaratne, T. 2001. "National Sample of Adults' Beliefs About Genetic Bases to Race and Gender." Unpublished raw data. Department of Psychology, University of Michigan.

Johnson, C. N. 1990. "If You Had My Brain, Where Would I Be? Children's Understanding of the Brain and Identity." *Child Development* 61: 962–972.

———. 2000. "Putting Things Together: The Development of Metaphysical Thinking." In K. S. Rosengren, C. N. Johnson, and L. Harris, eds., *Imagining the Impossible: Magical, Scientific, and Religious Thinking in Children.* New York: Cambridge University Press.

Johnson, C. N., and M. G. Jacobs. 2001. "Enchanted Objects: How Positive Connections Transform Thinking About the Very Nature of Things." Poster presented at the meeting of the Society for Research in Child Development, April, Minneapolis, Minn.

Johnson, C. N., and H. M. Wellman. 1982. "Children's Developing Conceptions of the Mind and Brain." *Child Development* 52: 222–234.

Johnson, M. 1993. *Moral Imagination: Implications of Cognitive Science for Ethics.* Chicago: University of Chicago Press.

Johnson, S., V. Slaughter, and S. Carey. 1998. "Whose Gaze Will Infants Follow? The Elicitation of Gaze Following in 12-Month-Olds." *Developmental Science* 1: 233–238.

Julius, A. 2002. *Transgressions: The Offenses of Art.* Chicago: University of Chicago Press.

Kagan, J. 1981. *The Second Year.* Cambridge, Mass.: Harvard University Press.

———. 1984. *The Nature of the Child.* New York: Basic Books.

Kahan, D. M. 1999. "The Progressive Appropriation of Disgust." In S. A. Bandes, ed., *The Passions of Law.* New York: New York University Press.

Kaiser, M. K., J. Jonides, and J. Alexander. 1986. "Intuitive Reasoning About Abstract and Familiar Physics Problems." *Memory and Cognition* 14: 308–312.

Kanner, L. 1943. "Autistic Disturbances of Affective Contact." *Nervous Child* 2: 217–250.

Kass, L. R. 1994. *The Hungry Soul.* New York: Free Press.

———. 2001. "Preventing a Brave New World: Why We Should Ban Human Cloning Now." *The New Republic,* May 21.

Keil, F. C. 1989. *Concepts, Kinds, and Cognitive Development.* Cambridge, Mass.: MIT Press.

———. 2004. "Developmental Psychology." Unpublished manuscript. Department of Psychology, Yale University.

Kelemen, D. 1996. "The Nature and Development of the Teleological Stance." Ph.D. dissertation, University of Arizona.

———. 1999a. "The Scope of Teleological Thinking in Preschool Children." *Cognition* 70: 241–272.

———. 1999b. "Why Are Rocks Pointy? Children's Preference for Teleological Explanations of the Natural World." *Developmental Psychology* 35: 1440–1453.

———. 1999c. "Function, Goals, and Intention: Children's Teleological Reasoning About Objects." *Trends in Cognitive Sciences* 12: 461–468.

Kelley, C. M., and L. L. Jacoby. 1996. "Adult Egocentrism: Subjective Experience Versus Analytic Bases for Judgment." *Journal of Memory and Language* 35: 157–175.

Kellman, J., and E. S. Spelke. 1983 "Perception of Partly Occluded Objects in Infancy." *Cognitive Psychology* 15: 483–524.

Kemler-Nelson, D. G. 1999. "Attention to Functional Properties in Toddlers' Naming and Problem-Solving." *Cognitive Development* 14: 77–100.

Kemler-Nelson, D. G., A. Frankenfield, C. Morris, and E. Blair. 2000a. "Young Children's Use of Functional Information to Categorize Artifacts: Three Factors That Matter." *Cognition* 77: 133–168.

Kemler-Nelson, D. G., R. Russell, N. Duke, and K. Jones. 2000b. "Two-Year-Olds Will Name Artifacts by Their Functions." *Child Development* 71: 1271–1288.

Kemler-Nelson, D. G., and 11 Swarthmore College Students. 1995. "Principle-Based Inferences in Young Children's Categorization: Revisiting the Impact of Function on the Naming of Artifacts." *Cognitive Development* 10: 347–380.

Keysar, B. 1994. "The Illusion of Transparency of Intention: Linguistic Perspective Taking in Text." *Cognitive Psychology* 26: 165–208.

Klin, A. 2000. "Attributing Social Meaning to Ambiguous Visual Stimuli in Higher Functioning Autism and Asperger Syndrome: The Social Attribution Task." *Journal of Child Psychology and Psychiatry* 41: 831–846.

Klin, A., W. Jones, R. Schultz, F. R. Volkmar, and D. J. Cohen. 2002. "Visual Fixation Patterns During Viewing of Naturalistic Social Situations as Predictors of Social Competence in Individuals with Autism." *Archives of General Psychiatry* 59: 809–816.

Koestler, A. 1964. *The Act of Creation.* New York: Dell.

Kornblith, H. 1993. *Inductive Inference and Its Natural Ground: An Essay in Naturalistic Epistemology.* Cambridge, Mass.: MIT Press.

Kripke, S. 1971. "Identity and Necessity." In M. K. Munitz, ed., *Identity and Individuation.* New York: New York University Press.

———. 1980. *Naming and Necessity.* Cambridge, Mass.: Harvard University Press.

Kuhlmeier, V., K. Wynn, and P. Bloom. 2003. "Attribution of Dispositional States by 12-Month-Olds." *Psychological Science* 14: 402–408.

Kurzweil, R. 1999. *The Age of Spiritual Machines: When Computers Exceed Human Intelligence*. New York: Penguin.

Lakoff, G. 1987. *Women, Fire, and Dangerous Things*. Chicago: University of Chicago Press.

Lazar, A., and J. Torney-Purta. 1991. "The Development of the Subconcepts of Death in Young Children: A Short-Term Longitudinal Study." *Cognitive Development* 62: 1321–1333.

Leach, P. 1989. *Your Baby and Child: From Birth to Age Five*. New York: Knopf.

Leslie, A. M. 1982. "The Perception of Causality in Infants." *Perception* 11, 173–186.

———. 1987. "Pretense and Representation: The Origins of 'Theory of Mind.'" *Psychological Review* 94: 412–426.

———. 1994a. "ToMM, ToBy, and Agency: Core Architecture and Domain Specificity." In L. Hirschfeld and S. Gelman, eds., *Mapping the Mind: Domain Specificity in Cognition and Culture*. New York: Cambridge University Press.

———. 1994b. "Pretending and Believing: Issues in the Theory of ToMM." *Cognition* 50: 193–200.

Lessing, A. 1983. "What Is Wrong with a Forgery?" In D. Dutton, ed., *The Forger's Art: Forgery and the Philosophy of Art*. University of California Press: Berkeley and Los Angeles.

Levi, P. 1988. *The Drowned and the Saved*. London: Abacus.

Levinson, J. 1979. "Defining Art Historically." *British Journal of Aesthetics* 19: 232–250.

———. 1989. "Refining Art Historically." *Journal of Aesthetics and Art Criticism* 47: 21–33.

———. 1993. "Extending Art Historically." *Journal of Aesthetics and Art Criticism* 51: 411–423.

Lewin, R. 1980. "Is Your Brain Really Necessary?" *Science* 210: 1232–1234.

Lewis, M. 2000a. "Self-conscious Emotions: Embarrassment, Pride, Shame, and Guilt." In M. Lewis and J. Haviland-Jones, eds., *Handbook of Emotions*. 2nd edition. New York: Guilford Press.

———. 2000b. "The Emergence of Human Emotions." In M. Lewis and J. Haviland-Jones, eds., *Handbook of Emotions*. 2nd edition. New York: Guilford Press.

Lewontin, R. 1972. "The Apportionment of Human Diversity." *Evolutionary Biology* 6: 381–398.

Lifton, R. J. 1986. *The Nazi Doctors: Medical Killing and the Psychology of Genocide*. New York: Basic Books.

Lillard, A. S. 1996. "Body or Mind: Children's Understanding of Pretense." *Child Development* 67: 1717–1734.

———. 1998. "Ethnopsychologies: Cultural Variations in Theories of Mind." *Psychological Bulletin* 123: 3–32.

Lithwick, D. 2002. "Habeas Corpses: What Are the Rights of Dead People?" Slate.com, http://slate.msn.com/id/20632222/.

Locke, J. 1947 [1690]. *An Essay Concerning Human Understanding*. New York: E. Dutton.

Lutz, D. 2003. "Young Children's Understanding of the Biological and Behavioral Processes Underlying Life and Death." Ph.D. dissertation, Department of Psychology, Yale University.

Lyas, C. 1997. *Aesthetics*. London: UCL Press.

Macnamara, J. 1982. *Names for Things: A Study of Human Learning*. Cambridge, Mass.: MIT Press.

Malt, B. C. 1991. "Word Meaning and Word Use." In P. Schwanenflugel, ed., *The Psychology of Word Meanings*. Hillsdale, N.J.: Erlbaum.

Marr, D. 1982. *Vision*. San Francisco: W. H. Freeman.

Martin, G. B., and R. D. Clark. 1982. "Distress Crying in Infants: Species and Peer Specificity." *Developmental Psychology* 18: 3–9.

Maynard Smith, J. 1964. "Group Selection and Kin Selection." *Nature* 201: 1145–1147.

Mayr, E. 1982. *The Growth of Biological Thought*. Cambridge, Mass.: Harvard University Press.

———. 1991. *One Long Argument: Charles Darwin and the Genesis of Modern Evolutionary Thought*. Cambridge, Mass.: Harvard University Press.

McCloskey, M., A. Caramazza, and B. Green. 1980. "Curvilinear Motion in the Absence of External Forces: Naïve Beliefs About the Motion of Objects." *Science* 210: 1139–1141.

McEwan, I. 2002. *Atonement*. New York: Doubleday.

McGinn, C. 1979. "Evolution, Animals, and the Basis of Morality." *Inquiry* 22: 92–98. Reprinted in P. Singer, ed., *Ethics*. New York: Oxford University Press.

McHugo, G. J., J. T. Lanzetta, D. G. Sullivan, R. D. Masters, and B. G. Englis. 1985. "Emotional Reactions to a Political Leader's Expressive Displays." *Journal of Personality and Social Psychology* 49: 1513–1529.

McWhorter, J. 2002. *The Power of Babel: A Natural History of Language*. New York: Freeman.

Medin, D. 1989. "Concepts and Conceptual Structure." *American Psychologist* 44: 1469–81.

Medin, D., and Ortony. A. 1989. "Psychological Essentialism." In S. Vosniadou and A. Ortony, eds., *Similarity and Analogical Reasoning*. Cambridge: Cambridge University Press.

Meltzoff, A. N., and M. K. Moore, 1977. "Imitations of Facial and Manual Gestures by Human Neonates." *Science* 198: 75–78.

———. 1983. "Newborn Infants Imitate Adult Facial Gestures." *Child Development* 54: 702–709.

Melzack, R., and D. Wall. 1983. *The Challenge of Pain*. New York: Basic Books.

Menand, L. 2002. "What Comes Naturally: Does Evolution Explain Who We Are?" *The New Yorker*, November 25, 96–101.

Miller, W. I. 1997. *The Anatomy of Disgust*. Cambridge, Mass.: Harvard University Press.

———. 1998. "Sheep, Joking, Cloning, and the Uncanny." In M. C. Nussbaum and C. R. Sunstein, eds., *Clones and Clones: Facts and Fantasies About Human Cloning*. New York: Norton.

Mineka, S., and M. Cook. 1993. "Mechanisms Involved in the Observational Conditioning of Fear." *Journal of Experimental Psychology: General* 122: 23–38.

Mischel, W., and E. B. Ebbesen. 1970. "Attention in Delay of Gratification." *Journal of Personality and Social Psychology* 16: 239–337.

Morris, M. W., and K. Peng. 1994. "Culture and Cause: American and Chinese Attributions for Social and Physical Events." *Journal of Personality and Social Psychology* 67: 949–971.

Murphy, G. L. 2002. *The Big Book of Concepts.* Cambridge, Mass.: MIT Press.

Murphy, G. L., and D. L. Medin. 1985. "The Role of Theories in Conceptual Coherence." *Psychological Review* 92: 289–316.

Murray, L., and C. Trevarthen. 1985. "Emotional Regulation of Interactions Between Two-Month-Olds and Their Mothers." In T. M. Field and N. A. Fox, eds., *Social Perception in Infants.* Norwood, N.J.: Ablex.

Naimark, N. M. 2001. *Fires of Hatred: Ethnic Cleansing in Twentieth-Century Europe.* Cambridge, Mass.: Harvard University Press.

Nemeroff, C., and P. Rozin. 1992. "Sympathetic Magical Beliefs and Kosher Dietary Practice: The Interaction of Rules and Feelings." *Ethos* 20: 96–115.

———. 1994. "The Contagion Concept in Adult Thinking in the United States: Transmission of Germs and Interpersonal Influence." *Ethos* 22: 158–186.

———. 2000. "The Makings of the Magical Mind." In K. S. Rosengren, C. N. Johnson, and L. Harris, eds., *Imagining the Impossible: Magical, Scientific, and Religious Thinking in Children.* New York: Cambridge University Press.

Newport, E. 1990. "Maturational Constraints on Language Learning." *Cognitive Science* 14: 11–28.

Ninio, A., and J. Bruner. 1978. "The Achievement and Antecedents of Labeling." *Journal of Child Language* 5: 1–15.

Nisbett, R. E., K. Peng, I. Choi, and A. Norenzayan. 2001. "Culture and Systems of Thought: Holistic Versus Analytic Cognition." *Psychological Review* 108: 291–310.

Norman, D. A. 1989. *The Design of Everyday Things.* New York: Doubleday.

Nucci, L., and E. Turiel. 1993. "God's Word, Religious Rules, and Their Relation to Christian and Jewish Children's Concepts of Morality." *Child Development* 64: 1485–1491.

Nussbaum, M. C. 1999. "'Secret Sewers of Vice': Disgust, Bodies, and the Law." In S. A. Bandes, ed., *The Passions of Law.* New York: New York University Press.

———. 2001. *Upheavals of Thought: The Intelligence of Emotions.* New York: Cambridge University Press.

Nussbaum, M. C., and J. Cohen, eds. 2002. *For Love of Country?* Boston, Mass.: Beacon Press.

O'Brien, T. 1990. *The Things They Carried.* New York: Broadway Books.

Pagels, E. 1979. *The Gnostic Gospels.* New York: Random House.

Paley, W. 1828. *Natural Theology.* 2nd edition. Oxford: J. Vincent.

Perner, J. 1991. *Understanding the Representational Mind.* Cambridge, Mass.: MIT Press.

Perner, J., S. Leekam, and H. Wimmer. 1987. "Three-Year-Olds' Difficulty with False Belief: The Case for a Conceptual Deficit." *British Journal of Developmental Psychology* 5: 125–137.

Peryam, D. R. 1963. "The Acceptance of Novel Foods." *Food Technology* 17: 33–39.

Petroski, H. 1993. *The Evolution of Useful Things.* New York: Knopf.

Pettigrew, T. F. 1998. "Intergroup Contact Theory." *Annual Review of Psychology* 49: 65–85.

Pettigrew, T. F., and L. R. Tropp. 2000. "Does Intergroup Contact Reduce Prejudice? Recent Meta-analytic Findings." In S. Oskamp, ed., *Reducing Prejudice and Discrimination.* Mahwah, N.J.: Erlbaum.

Piaget, J. 1929. *The Child's Conception of the World.* New York: Harcourt.

———. 1954. *The Construction of Reality in the Child.* New York: Basic Books.

Pinker, S. 1994. *The Language Instinct.* New York: HarperCollins.

———. 1997. *How the Mind Works.* New York: Norton.

———. 2002. *The Blank Slate: The Denial of Human Nature in Modern Intellectual Life.* New York: Norton.

Pinker, S., and P. Bloom. 1990. "Natural Language and Natural Selection." *Behavioral and Brain Sciences* 13: 707–784.

Pizarro, D. 2000. "Nothing More Than Feelings? The Role of Emotions in Moral Judgment." *Journal for the Theory of Social Behavior* 30: 355–375.

Pizarro, D., and P. Bloom. 2002. "The Intelligence of the Moral Emotions: Comment on Haidt 2001." *Psychological Review* 110: 193–196.

Polkinghorne, J. C. 1999. *Belief in God in an Age of Science.* New Haven: Yale University Press.

Posner, R. 1992. *Sex and Reason.* Cambridge, Mass.: Harvard University Press.

Postman, N. 1982. *The Disappearance of Childhood.* New York: Random House.

Povinelli, D. J., J. E. Reaux, D. T. Bierschwale, A. D. Allain, and B. B. Simon. 1997. "Exploitation of Pointing as a Referential Gesture in Young Children, but Not Adolescent Chimpanzees." *Cognitive Development* 12: 327–365.

Povinelli, D. J., and J. Vonk. 2003. "Chimpanzee Minds: Suspiciously Human?" *Trends in Cognitive Sciences* 7: 157–160.

Powers, S. 2002. *A Problem from Hell.* New York: Basic Books.

Preissler, M. A. 2003. "Symbolic Understanding of Pictures and Words in Low-Functioning Children with Autism and Normally Developing 18- and 24-Month-Old Toddlers." Ph.D. dissertation, New York University.

Preissler, M. A., and S. Carey. Under review. "Do Both Pictures and Words Function as Symbols for 18- and 24-Month-Old Children?"

Premack, D., and A. J. Premack. 1997. "Infants Assign Value to the Goal-Directed Actions of Self-Propelled Objects." *Journal of Cognitive Neuroscience* 9: 848–856.

Proffitt, D. L., and D. L. Gilden. 1989. "Understanding Natural Dynamics." *Journal of Experimental Psychology: Human Perception and Performance* 15: 384–393.

Provine, R. R. 2000. *Laughter: A Scientific Investigation.* New York: Viking.

Putnam, H. 1973. "Meaning and Reference." *The Journal of Philosophy* 70: 699–711.

———. 1975a. "The Meaning of 'Meaning.'" In H. Putnam, ed., *Mind, Language, and Reality.* New York: Cambridge University Press.

————. 1975b. "Philosophy and Our Mental Life." In H. Putnam, ed., *Mind, Language, and Reality*. New York: Cambridge University Press.

Rafal, R. 1997. "Balint Syndrome." In T. E. Feinberg and M. J. Farah, eds., *Behavioral Neurology and Neuropsychology*. New York: McGraw-Hill.

————. 1998. "Neglect." In R. Parasuraman, ed., *The Attentive Brain*. Cambridge, Mass.: MIT Press.

Ramachandran, V. S., and S. Blakeslee. 1998. *Phantoms in the Brain: Probing the Mysteries of the Human Mind*. New York: William Morrow.

Ramachandran, V. S., and W. Hirstein. 1999. "The Science of Art." *Journal of Consciousness Studies* 6–7: 15–41.

Rawls, J. A. 1971. *A Theory of Justice*. Cambridge, Mass.: Harvard University Press.

Reddy, V. 2000. "Coyness in Early Infancy." *Developmental Science* 3: 186–192.

Reé, J. 2002. "Francine-Machine." *London Review of Books,* May 9, 16–18.

Regolin, L., and G. Vallortigara. 1995. "Perception of Partly Occluded Objects by Young Chicks." *Perception and Psychophysics* 57: 971–976.

Repacholi, B. M., and A. Gopnik. 1997. "Early Reasoning About Desires: Evidence from 14- and 18-Month-Olds." *Developmental Psychology* 33: 12–21.

Reza, Y. 1996. *Art*. Trans. C. Hampton. London: Faber & Faber.

Rochat, P. T. 2001. *The Infant's World*. Cambridge, Mass.: Harvard University Press.

Rochat, P., T. Morgan, and M. Carpenter. 1997. "Young Children's Sensitivity to Movement Information Specifying Social Causality." *Cognitive Development* 12: 441–465.

Rosenberg, H. 1973. *The Anxious Object: Art Today and Its Audience*. New York: Macmillan.

Roth, D., and A. M. Leslie. 1998. "Solving Belief Problems: Towards a Task Analysis." *Cognition* 66: 1–31.

Rozin, P. 1986. "One-Trial Acquired Likes and Dislikes in Humans: Disgust as a US, Food Predominance, and Negative Learning Predominance." *Learning and Motivation* 17: 180–189.

Rozin, P., and A. Fallon. 1987. "A Perspective on Disgust. *Psychological Review* 94: 23–41.

Rozin, P., J. Haidt, C. R. McCauley, and S. Imada. 1997. "Disgust: Preadaptation and the Cultural Evolution of a Food-Based Emotion." In H. Macbeth, ed., *Food Preferences and Taste: Continuity and Change*. Providence: Berghahn Books.

Rozin, P., J. Haidt, and C. R. McCauley. 2000. "Disgust." In M. Lewis and J. M. Haviland-Jones, eds., *Handbook of Emotions*. 2nd edition. New York: Guilford Press.

Rozin, P., L. Hammer, H. Oster, T. Horowitz, and V. Marmora. 1986. "The Child's Conception of Food: Differentiation of Categories of Rejected Substances in the 1.4 to 5 Year Age Range." *Appetite* 7: 141–151.

Rozin, P., L. Millman, and C. Nemeroff. 1986. "Operation of the Laws of Sympathetic Magic in Disgust and Other Domains." *Journal of Personality and Social Psychology* 50: 703–712.

Russo, R. 2001. *Empire Falls*. New York: Random House.

Sacks, O. 1995. *An Anthropologist on Mars*. New York: Knopf.

Sagi, A., and M. L. Hoffman. 1976. "Empathetic Distress in the Newborn." *Developmental Psychology* 12: 175–176.

Saint-Exupéry, A. de. 1943. *The Little Prince.* New York: Harcourt.

Saletan, W. 2001. "Shag the Dog." Slate.com, http://slate.msn.com/FrameGame/entires/01–01–04_103801.as

Salovey, P., J. D. Mayer, and D. Caruso. 2002. "The Positive Psychology of Emotional Intelligence." In C. R. Snyder and S. J. Lopez, eds., *The Handbook of Positive Psychology.* New York: Oxford University Press.

Schelling, T. C. 1984. *Choice and Consequence: Perspectives of an Errant Economist.* Cambridge, Mass.: Harvard University Press.

Schneider, E. 1999. *Discovering My Autism: Apologia Pro Vita Sua with Apologies to Cardinal Newman.* London: Jessica Kingsley.

Shaw, L. L., C. D. Batson, and R. M. Todd. 1994. "Empathy Avoidance: Forestalling Feeling for Another in Order to Escape the Motivational Consequences." *Journal of Personality and Social Psychology* 67: 879–887.

Sheets, H. M. 2000. "Baffled, Bewildered—and Smitten: How to Learn to Stop Worrying and Love the Art You Don't Understand." *ARTnews,* September, 130–134.

Shepard, R. 1990. *Mind Sights: Original Visual Illusions, Ambiguities, and Other Anomalies.* New York: W. H. Freeman.

Shermer, M. 2000. *How We Believe: The Search for God in an Age of Science.* New York: Freeman.

———. 2003. "Digits and Fidgets: Is the Universe Fine-Tuned for Life?" *Scientific American,* January, 35.

Shweder, R. A. 1994. "Are Moral Intuitions Self-evident Truths?" *Criminal Justice Ethics* 13: 24-23.

Siegal, M. 1995. "Becoming Mindful of Food and Conversation." *Current Directions in Psychological Science* 6: 177–181.

Siegal, M., and D. L. Share. 1990, "Contamination Sensitivity in Young Children." *Developmental Psychology* 26: 455–458.

Siegal, M., and C. C. Peterson. 1996. "Breaking the Mold: A Fresh Look at Children's Understanding of Questions About Lies and Mistakes." *Developmental Psychology* 32: 322–334.

Sigman, M. D., C. Kasari, J.-H. Kwon, and N. Yirmiya. 1992. "Responses to the Negative Emotions of Others by Autistic, Mentally Retarded, and Normal Children." *Child Development* 63: 796–807.

Simmer, M. L. 1971. "Newborns' Response to the Cry of Another Infant." *Developmental Psychology* 5: 136–150.

Singer, D. G., and J. L. Singer. 1990. *The House of Make-believe: Children's Play and Developing Imagination.* Cambridge, Mass.: Harvard University Press.

Singer, P. 1981. *The Expanding Circle: Ethics and Sociobiology.* New York: Farrar Straus Giroux.

———. 2000. "The Good Life." In *Writings on an Ethical Life.* New York: HarperCollins.

———. 2001. "Heavy Petting." Nerve.com, http//www.nerve.com/Opinions/Singer/heavyPetting/main.as

Slater, A., and C. Quinn, C. 2001. "Face Recognition in the Newborn Infant." *Infant and Child Development* 10: 21–24.

Slaughter, V., R. Jaakkola, and S. Carey. 1999. "Constructing a Coherent Theory: Children's Biological Understanding of Life and Death." In M. Siegal and C. C. Peterson, eds., *Children's Understanding of Biology and Health*. New York: Cambridge University Press.

Smith, A. 1976 [1759]. *A Theory of the Moral Sentiments*. Indianapolis: Liberty Classics.

Smuts, B. 1999. Untitled essay. In A. Gutmann, ed., *The Lives of Animals*. Princeton: Princeton University Press.

Sober, E. 1994. *From a Biological Point of View*. New York: Cambridge University Press.

Sober, E., and D. S. Wilson. 1998. *Unto Others: The Evolution and Psychology of Unselfish Behavior*. Cambridge, Mass.: Harvard University Press.

Solomon, R. C. 1999. "Peter Singer's Expanding Circle: Compassion and the Liberation of Ethics." In D. Jamieson, ed., *Singer and His Critics*. Cambridge, Mass.: Blackwell.

Spelke, E. S. 1994. "Initial Knowledge: Six Suggestions." *Cognition* 50: 443–447.

———. 2003. "What Makes Humans Smart?" In D. Gentner and S. Goldin-Meadow, eds., *Advances in the Investigation of Language and Thought*. Cambridge, Mass.: MIT Press.

Spelke, E. S., K. Breinlinger, K. Jacobson, and A. Phillips. 1993. "Gestalt Relations and Object Perception: A Developmental Study." *Perception* 22: 1483–1501.

Spelke, E. S., R. Kestenbaum, D. J. Simons, and D. Wein. 1995. "Spatiotemporal Continuity, Smoothness of Motion and Object Identity in Infancy." *British Journal of Developmental Psychology* 13: 113–143.

Spelke, E. S., A. Phillips,, and A. L. Woodward. 1995. "Infant's Knowledge of Object Motion and Human Action." In D. Sperber, D. Premack, and A. J. Premack, eds., *Causal Cognition*. New York: Oxford University Press.

Sperber, D. 1996. *Explaining Culture: A Naturalistic Approach*. Oxford: Blackwell.

Stengel, R. 2000. *You're Too Kind: A Brief History of Flattery*. New York: Simon & Schuster.

Sterelny, K. 2001. *Dawkins vs. Gould: Survival of the Fittest*. New York: Totem Books.

Sternberg, R. J. 2001. "A Duplex Theory of Hate and Its Application to Massacres and Genocides." Unpublished manuscript. Department of Psychology, Yale University.

Strack, F., L. L. Martin, and S. Stepper. 1988. "Inhibiting and Facilitating Conditions of the Human Smile: A Nonobtrusive Test of the Facial Feedback Hypothesis." *Journal of Personality and Social Psychology* 54: 768–776.

Subbotsky, E. V. 1993. *Foundations of the Mind*. Cambridge, Mass.: Harvard University Press.

Sully, J. 1896. *Studies of Childhood*. New York: D. Appleton and Co.

Sylvia, C., and W. Novak. 1997. *A Change of Heart*. Boston: Little Brown.

Taylor, M. 1999. *Imaginary Companions and the Children Who Create Them*. New York: Oxford University Press.

Taylor, T. 2002. *The Buried Soul: How Humans Invented Death*. London: Fourth Estate.

Templeton, A. R. 1998. "Human Races: A Genetic and Evolutionary Perspective." *American Anthropologist* 100: 632–650.

Termine, N. T., and C. E. Izard. 1988. "Infants' Response to Their Mother's Expressions of Joy and Sadness." *Developmental Psychology* 24: 223–229.

Tetlock, P. E., O. V. Kristel, B. Elson, M. C. Green, and J. Lerner. 2000. "The Psychology of the Unthinkable: Taboo Trade-offs, Forbidden Base Rates, and Heretical Counterfactuals." *Journal of Personality and Social Psychology* 78: 853–870.

Thomas, G. V., R. Nye, and E. J. Robinson. 1994. "How Children View Pictures: Children's Responses to Pictures as Things in Themselves and as Representations of Something Else." *Cognitive Development* 9: 141–164.

Tomasello, M. 1998. "Uniquely Primate, Uniquely Human." *Developmental Science* 1: 1–16.

Tomasello, M., J. Call, and B. Hare. 2003. "Chimpanzees Understand Psychological States—the Question Is Which Ones and to What Extent." *Trends in Cognitive Sciences* 7: 153–156.

Trivers, R. L. 1971. "The Evolution of Reciprocal Altruism." *Quarterly Review of Biology* 46: 35–57.

———. 1985. *Social Evolution*. Reading, Mass.: Benjamin/Cummings.

Tronick, E. Z., H. Als, L. Adamson, S. Wise, and T. B. Brazelton. 1978. "The Infant's Response to Entrapment Between Contradictory Messages." *Journal of the American Academy of Child and Adolescent Psychiatry* 17: 1–13.

Turiel, E. 1998. "The Development of Morality." In W. Damon, series ed., *Handbook of Child Psychology*. Vol. 3, N. Eisenberg, volume ed., *Social, Emotional, and Personality Development*. New York: Wiley.

Turiel, E., and K. Neff. 2000. "Religion, Culture and Beliefs About Reality in Moral Reasoning." In K. S. Rosengren, C. N. Johnson, and L. Harris, eds., *Imagining the Impossible: Magical, Scientific, and Religious Thinking in Children*. New York: Cambridge University Press.

de Waal, F. 1996. *Good Natured: The Origins of Right and Wrong in Humans and Other Animals*. Cambridge, Mass.: Harvard University Press.

Walker [Jeyifous], S. 1992. "Supernatural Beliefs, Natural Kinds, and Conceptual Structure." *Memory and Cognition* 20: 655–662.

Walker-Andrews, A. S. 1997. "Infants' Perception of Expressive Behavior: Differentiation of Multimodal Information." *Psychological Bulletin* 121: 437–456.

Wallace, A. R. 1889. *Darwinism*. London: Macmillan.

Warburton, N. 2003. *The Art Question*. New York: Routledge.

Ward, T. B., A. H. Becker, S. D. Hass, and E. Vela, 1991. "Attribute Availability and the Shape Bias in Children's Category Construction." *Cognitive Development* 6: 143–167.

Wegner, D. 2002. *The Illusion of Conscious Will*. Cambridge, Mass.: MIT Press.

Wellman, H. M. 1990. *The Child's Theory of Mind*. Cambridge, Mass.: MIT Press.

Wellman, H. M., D. Cross, and J. Watson. 2001. "Meta-analysis of Theory-Of-Mind Development: The Truth About False Belief." *Child Development* 72: 655–684.

Wellman, H. M., and D. Estes. 1986. "Early Understanding of Mental Entities: A Reexamination of Childhood Realism." *Child Development* 57: 910–923.

Wells, G. L., and R. E. Petty. 1980. "The Effects of Overt Head Movement on Persuasion: Compatibility and Incompatibility Responses." *Basic and Applied Social Psychology* 1: 219–230.

Werner, H., and H. Kaplan. 1963. *Symbol Formation*. New York: Wiley.

Werness, H. B. 1983. "*Han van Meegeren* fecit." In D. Dutton, ed., *The Forger's Art: Forgery and the Philosophy of Art*. Berkeley and Los Angeles: University of California Press.

West, R., and R. Young. 2002. "Do Domestic Dogs Show Any Evidence of Being Able to Count?" *Animal Cognition* 5: 183–186.

White, R. 1993. "Technological and Social Dimensions of 'Aurignacian-Age' Body Ornaments Across Europe." In H. Knecht, A. Pike-Tay, and R. White, eds., *Before Lascaux: The Complete Record of the Upper Paleolithic*. Boca Raton, Fla.: CRC Press.

Wilkinson, G. S. 1984. "Reciprocal Food Sharing in the Vampire Bat." *Nature* 308: 181–184.

Willett, W. C. 2001. *Eat, Drink, and Be Healthy*. New York: Simon & Schuster.

Williams, G. C. 1966. *Adaptation and Natural Selection: A Critique of Some Current Evolutionary Thought*. Princeton: Princeton University Press.

Wills, G. 1999. *Saint Augustine*. New York: Penguin.

Wilson, R. A. 1999. "The Individual in Biology and Psychology." In V. G. Hardcastle, ed., *Where Biology Meets Psychology: Philosophical Essays*. Cambridge, Mass.: MIT Press.

Wilson, T. D, and N. C. Brekke. 1994. "Mental Contamination and Mental Correction: Unwanted Influences on Judgments and Evaluations." *Psychological Bulletin* 116: 117–142.

Wimmer, H., and J. Perner. 1983. "Beliefs About Beliefs: Representation and Constraining Function of Wrong Beliefs in Young Children's Understanding of Deception." *Cognition* 13: 103–128.

Wolfe, A. 2001. *Moral Freedom: The Search for Virtue in a World of Choice*. New York: Norton.

Wolfe, T. 1975. *The Painted Word*. New York: Bantam Books.

Wollheim, R. 1980. *Art and Its Objects*. New York: Cambridge University Press.

———. 1993. "Danto's Gallery of Indiscernibles." In M. Rollins, ed., *Danto and His Critics*. Cambridge, Mass.: Blackwell.

Wood, G. 2002. *Edison's Eve: A Magical History of the Quest for Mechanical Life*. New York: Knopf.

Woodward, A. L. 1998. "Infants Selectively Encode the Goal Object of an Actor's Reach." *Cognition* 69: 1–34.

Woolley, J. D. 2000. "The Development of Beliefs About Direct Mental-Physical Causation in Imagination, Magic, and Religion." In K. S. Rosengren, C. N. Johnson, and L. Harris, eds., *Imagining the Impossible: Magical, Scientific, and Religious Thinking in Children*. New York: Cambridge University Press.

Woolley, J. D., and K. E. Phelps. 1994. "Young Children's Practical Reasoning About Imagination." *British Journal of Developmental Psychology* 12: 53–67.

Woolley, J. D., and H. M. Wellman. 1990. "Young Children's Understanding of Realities, Nonrealities, and Appearances." *Child Development* 61: 946–961.

Wright, R. 1994. *The Moral Animal: Why We Are the Way We Are: The New Science of Evolutionary Psychology.* New York: Random House.

———. 2000. *NonZero: The Logic of Human Destiny.* New York: Pantheon Books.

Wynn, K. 1992. "Addition and Subtraction by Human Infants." *Nature* 358: 749–750.

———. 2000. "Findings of Addition and Subtraction Are Robust and Consistent: A Reply to Wakeley, Rivera, and Langer." *Child Development* 71: 1535–1536.

Wynn, K., and W.-C. Chiang. 1998. "Limits to Infants' Knowledge of Objects: The Case of Magical Appearance." *Psychological Science* 9: 448–455.

Xu, F., S. Carey, and J. Welch. 1999. "Infants' Ability to Use Object Kind Information for Object Individuation." *Cognition* 70: 137–166.

Yenawine, P. 1991. *How to Look at Modern Art.* New York: Harry N. Abrams.

Zahn-Waxler, C., and J. Robinson. 1995. "Empathy and Guilt: Early Origins of Feelings of Responsibility." In J. Tangney and K. W. Fischer, eds., *Self-conscious Emotions: The Psychology of Shame, Guilt, Embarrassment, and Pride.* New York: Guilford.

Zahn-Waxler, C., J. L. Robinson, and R. N. Emde. 1992. "The Development of Empathy in Twins." *Developmental Psychology* 28: 1038–1047.

INDEX